THE WORLD GYM

MUSCLEBUILDING SYSTEM

D1608903

THE WORLD GYM

MUSCLEBUILDING SYSTEM

JOE GOLD

WITH
ROBERT
KENNEDY

CONTEMPORARY
BOOKS, INC.
CHICAGO • NEW YORK

Library of Congress Cataloging-in-Publication Data

Gold, Joe.
   The World Gym musclebuilding system/Joe Gold with Robert Kennedy.
   p. cm.
   Cover subtitle: Learn the secrets to building hard muscle
   ISBN 0-8092-4713-5 (pbk.)
     1. Bodybuilding.   2. World Gym (Venice, LosAngeles, Calif.)
–Directories.   I. Kennedy, Robert, 1938–   II. Title.
GV546.5.G64 1987
646.7′5—dc19

Published by Contemporary Books, Inc.
180 North Michigan Avenue, Chicago, Illinois 60601
Manufactured in the United States of America
International Standard Book Number: 0-8092-4713-5

Published simultaneously in Canada by Beaverbooks, Ltd.
195 Allstate Parkway, Valleywood Business Park
Markham, Ontario L3R 4T8 Canada

CONTENTS

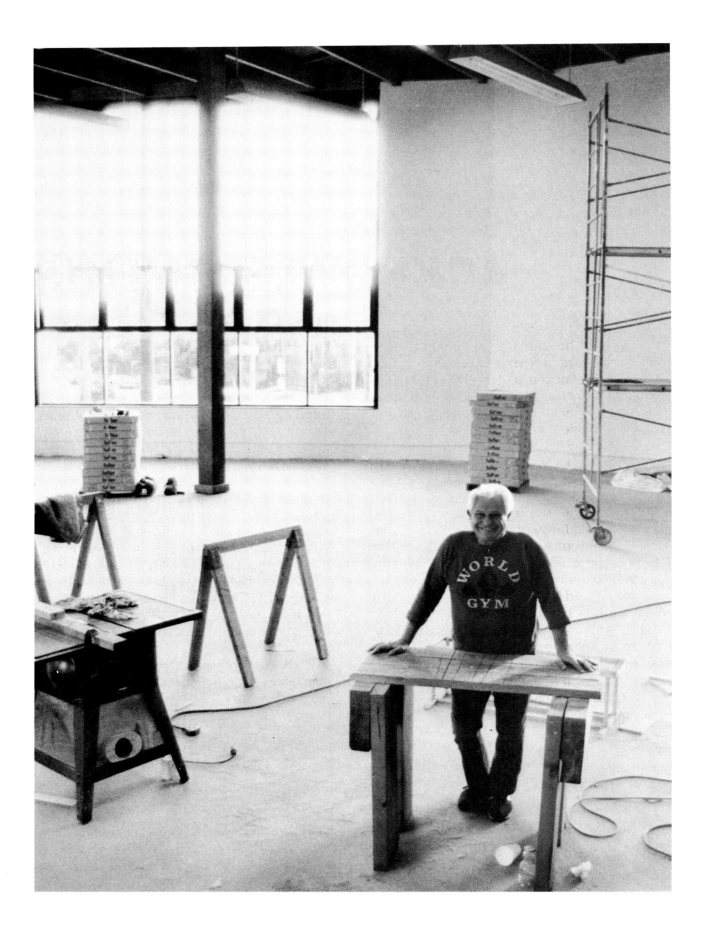

ACKNOWLEDGMENTS

I've said it before but it bears repeating. A book is always a combined effort. Clay Smudsky of Contemporary Books has to be thanked for his part in this production. I also owe a special debt of gratitude to Joe and Ben Weider, whose magazines *Flex*, *Muscle and Fitness*, *Shape*, and *Men's Fitness* keep bodybuilding hot! Year after year the IFBB goes from strength to strength.

To my friend Arnold Schwarzenegger, who wrote the foreword to this book, I owe more than I could put into words. Since day one when he first visited my gym in the late sixties he has been an inspiration in a thousand ways. What a wonderful friend he has been over the years.

Thanks to Robert Kennedy of *MuscleMag International* for helping me organize my thoughts on the original manuscript and to my copyeditor Al Simonaitis at Contemporary for keeping the writing lean and tight.

Of the photographers . . . super lensman Art Zeller took most of the quality pics within these pages. Art can do things with a camera that border on magic. Additional super photogs whom I would like to thank include Steve Douglas, Paula Crane, Bill Heimanson, Doris Barrilleaux, Chris Lund, Garry Barlett, Denie Walter, Walt Sorenson, Robert Nailon, Doug White, Monty Heron, Tapio Hautala, Bob Flippin, Peter Potter, Edward Hankey, Bob Gruskin, John Campos, Jim Marchand, Al Antuck, John Balik, Mike Neveaux, Reg Bradford, Wayne Gallasch, Paul Goode, Ken Korentayer, Glenn Low, Lou Parees, Roger Shelley, Bill Reynolds, Russ Warner, Eric Chapman, Andrea Lamantia, Geof Collins, and my custom photoprocessor, Mike Read.

And to the bodybuilding champions . . . I especially want to offer my gratitude. I hope we have truthfully depicted your muscles and your training intensity!

Dedicated to
Arnold
With a special thanks to all who have
been associated with World Gym.

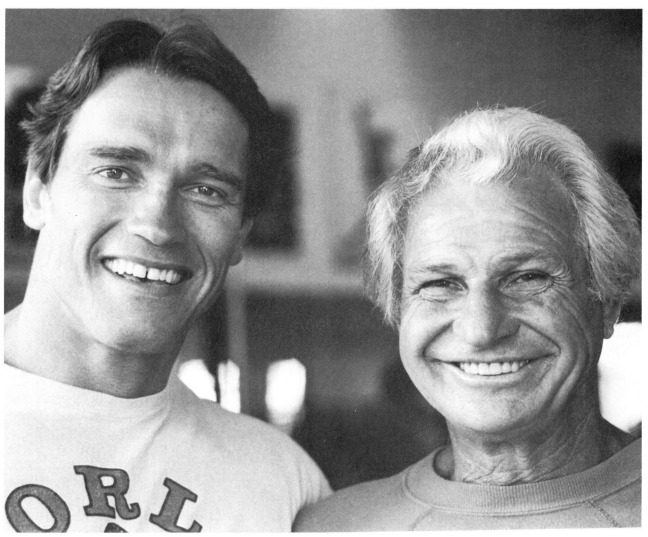
Arnold and Joe: the World never knew two closer friends.

FOREWORD

The friendship between me and Joe Gold is almost legendary. It's true. The feeling I have for Joe is hard to describe, but it is as solid and sure as my love for bodybuilding.

World Gym always felt like home to me, not a cold impersonal place like so many other facilities. Joe opened both his gym and his heart to me. He was not only generous to me, but always helped out-of-town or foreign bodybuilders by inviting them to a free workout.

Joe helped me in the beginning when I had nothing. He asked for nothing in return. Now that I am a success everyone is offering to help me—but it doesn't mean as much. What counts are those early kindnesses that were given from the heart, with no thought of self-gain. How can you forget a man who never charged you for gym membership? Who more than once spent the day's "take" on making sure that I had a decent meal after my evening workout? Joe looked after me when I needed it and couldn't repay his kindness. His support was always there, and always bathed in honesty. For example, he travelled to Australia in 1980 to support me in my bid for a seventh Mr. Olympia title. After the preliminary judging he told me: "Arnold, you're definitely in the top three! You have to be aggressive in the free posing and fight your way up." I

didn't like what I was hearing, but I took Joe's advice and pulled out all the stops. At the conclusion of the evening show, before the results were tabulated, Joe told me: "You've done it, you were magnificent. In my opinion, you've definitely won." He was right.

The man's become a kind of father figure to me, born out of my deep respect. Actually he and I are very different types. I pushed my way to the top of bodybuilding through brute determination and then used that same controlled, limitless energy to command success in the movie business. I knew what I wanted and went for it. Joe was always laid-back, never thinking about himself. He would come into the gym daily and stay. Unlike many gym owners who drop in only occasionally to check cash flow, Joe came to check the apparatus. Was a pulley in need of repair? Did the moving parts need oiling? Were the bushings wearing out? Because of my height a couple of his early machines were too small for me to use properly. The minute Joe found out, he set up his welding kit and made the adjustment. He never expected a "Thank you," but I appreciated his actions more than he will ever know.

Today when you go to World Gym you will find Joe there looking after the day-to-day business. It's that way because he

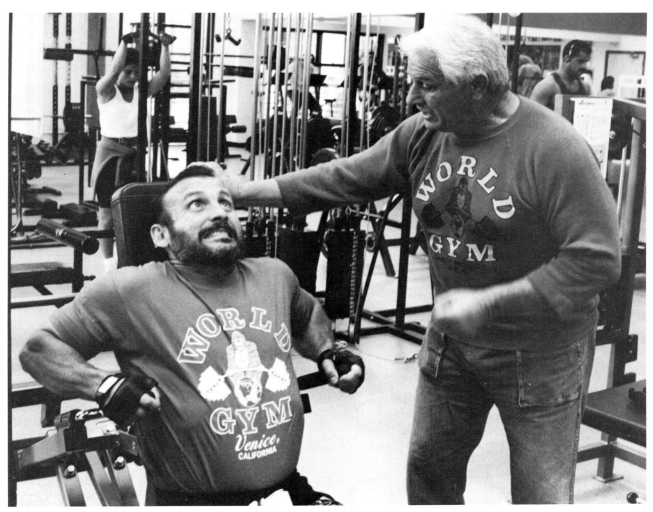

Joe gives a World Gym regular some advice.

cares. You have only to look at the gym, with its high ceilings, huge windows, and spacious outdoor training decks, to know that Joe Gold thinks of the bodybuilder's needs first when he designs a training establishment. I watched him and his team build this gym from the ground up, brick by brick, until in early 1987 it became a training paradise for the modern hard-core bodybuilding enthusiast.

When I first began bodybuilding as a hungry teenager in Austria I had to make do with a small, dark gym, set under the sports stadium in my hometown of Graz. It was the only place that had free weights. As I progressed, I visited and trained in scores of countries. No one has trained at more different gyms than I have. It's one of

the perks of being a bodybuilding champion. All the more reason my claim that the World Gym in Venice, California, is the supreme training environment should be taken seriously.

In 1968 I worked out at Joe's original hard-core gym on Pacific Avenue in Venice. I had sampled other establishments, but none suited my requirements. I needed light. I needed space. I needed sturdy, smooth-running equipment. This gym had everything. No one ever sat on a bench and read a newspaper at this gym. Idle gossip was invariably limited to a short, breathless sentence, a wink or a nod between sets. Members came to train their hearts out, not to socialize or waste time. I remember one early conversation with Joe in which he detailed how his pulleys should be set to maximize their smoothness. He knew what he was talking about—World Gym apparatus is silky-smooth from any angle, at any resistance. It's a joy to work with.

The gym quickly became my favorite place to exercise, and it has remained so ever since. My early workouts with Dave Draper are indelibly etched in my mind. They were followed by hundreds of super sweat-drenched sessions with Franco Columbu, Frank Zane, Ed Corney, Mike Katz, and scores of other top stars, all of whom regarded this gym as the best. Together, in this establishment, we lifted bodybuilding from obscurity to the public acceptance it enjoys today.

I still train at World's, usually around eight in the morning. The gym is known as the home of champions. The early birds

that I train alongside include Tom Platz, Lou Ferrigno, Bertil Fox, Bob Paris, Reg Park, Jusup Wilcosz, Rachel McLish, Franco Columbu, Samir Bannout, Brad Harris, Irvin Kozewski, Ali Malla, Ed Giuliani, and just about every established champion in our sport.

This book follows as a logical conclusion to the success of World Gym and its scores of franchised establishments. It dwells on quality training. It exudes concern for the bodybuilder. It inspires and informs with that magical touch of truth and sincerity that is synonymous with Joe himself. He is the original honest iron man, dedicated to his sport and to giving value for money. I trust him completely. He has never taken advantage of my name, nor has he ever used me to benefit himself.

Joe wrote this book in his own words. Read it through and you'll learn how to be

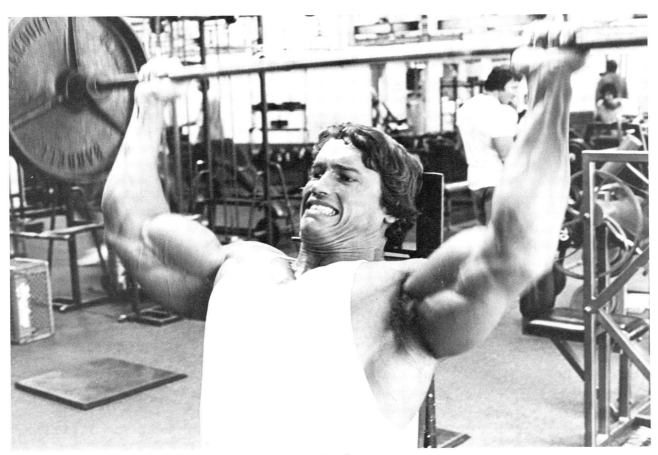
Arnold training at World Gym—an unbeatable combination.

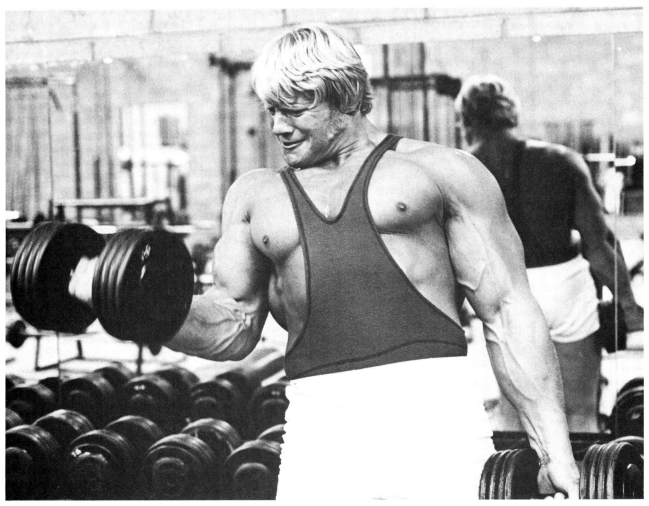

The legendary Dave Draper.

a better bodybuilder. Joe also tells you how to have more confidence, personal power, and zest for life.

Keep it handy in your bodybuilding library for those times when you need knowledge or inspiration. Joe's integrity and stubbornness in always seeking perfection shows through in this book. I heartily recommend this book to all who seek greatness. And that, Joe . . . is from the heart.

Arnold Schwarzenegger

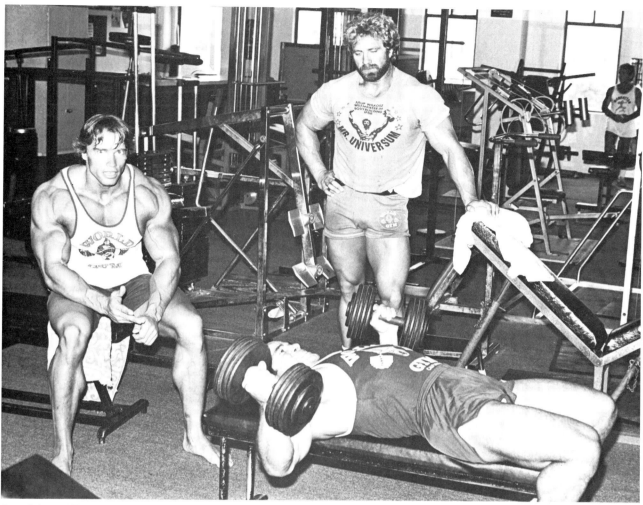

Arnold and Franco train at World under the watchful eye of Jusup Wilcosz.

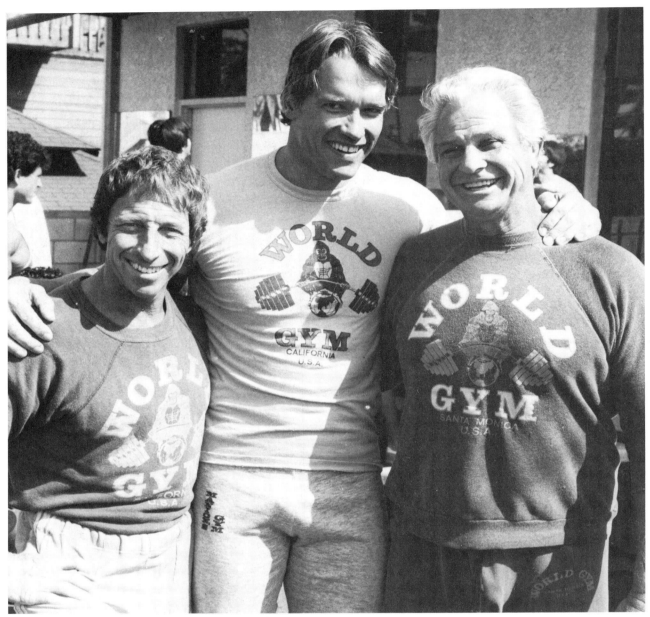

Eddie Giuliani, Arnold Schwarzenegger, and Joe Gold.

INTRODUCTION

HOW WORLD'S BECAME WORLD'S
AS TOLD BY EDDIE GIULIANI

It was 1967. Joe Weider had sent me a ticket to visit California for the Mr. Western America contest. The fact that I failed to win—placing third—didn't bother me a bit. I had seen Southern California and fallen in love. Two years later I returned to live there permanently. I was going to train in the Valley because many stars had come from that area, but Joe Weider told me to train at the new hard-core gym in Venice. The gym was run by a 45-year-old bodybuilding enthusiast named Joe Gold.

When I got to the place on Main Street, I was shocked. It was unlike any gym I had ever seen. The building was like a square box. There was not one picture of a bodybuilder on the walls. How many hard-core gyms have you seen without a single bodybuilding photo on display? There was no music in the gym. At that time Joe just didn't like the idea. And lastly, quite unbelievably, the gym had no name. There was no sign outside, no printed letters on the window, no name on the door. The only giveaway to hard-core enthusiasts trying to find the place was the sound of clanging iron, which reverberated into the street outside, unnoticed by most but music of the highest caliber to dedicated iron men.

The first person who was super nice to me at the gym was Zabo Kozewski. He had won every "best abs" award that he had entered, and he had entered plenty!

Dave Draper was the star of the gym in those days. His long golden hair attracted the hip audience. Most bodybuilders still had crew cuts and were getting typed as "square" gorillas with no brains. Bodybuilding was still considered a pretty insane pastime by the general public.

Joe Weider used Dave Draper time and again on his magazine covers. He sold more copies when the blond bomber displayed his wares. Dave actually pioneered early-morning training. He reasoned that the air was purer, there was less traffic, the mood was tranquil, and he could concentrate better. "The gym was ideally suited," he said, "to drumming up a pump!"

When Arnold crossed the Atlantic, quickly followed by Franco, a magic atmosphere crept into the gym. We all knew something special was happening. Art Zeller, the world's most patient photographer (and arguably the world's greatest),

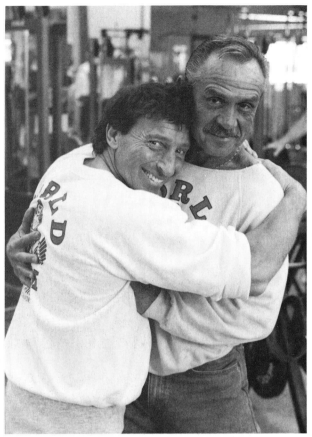

Eddie and good friend Irvin "Zabo" Kozewski.

talent—Frank Zane, Dave Draper, Franco Columbu, Arnold Schwarzenegger, Ed Corney, Zabo Kozewski, Mike Katz—I suddenly realized that virtually all the stars of bodybuilding had decided to train under one roof. The gym was a block from the Pacific Ocean. It was permeated with an unusual light that resulted from the sun streaming through the gym's frosted windows after bouncing off the white buildings across the street. The equipment was hard-core all the way. If Joe Gold thought it would make a better machine, he would triple up the amount of steel. Everything was precision-built. Even the handles of the dumbbells and pulleys fit the hand like a custom revolver. Arnold said, "When you train at Joe's gym all the machines run so smoothly, you can use 10 to 15 pounds more on all the exercises."

When the world found out about this gym we were inundated with people from all over. They came to check us out. More than that, they brought tape measures and Polaroid cameras and tried to copy everything. They went back home with their numbers, but to this day no one has been able to copy the equipment successfully. Joe's personal touch couldn't be duplicated. Like the famed Italian automobile designer Enzo Ferrari, he is one of a kind. Mass production never entered his mind.

The only thing that riles him is when the occasional member fails to show respect for the gym that Joe has put his heart into. He has an unwritten "one warning only" rule. Members who drop weights get an instant cash refund of their membership, accompanied by a forceful: "That's it, you're out!"

For the last decade and more, Zabo Kozewski and I have worked for World Gym. I'm up at six in the morning. It's easier in Southern California. The birds are up and singing and help you out of bed. When you sleep late in the morning you kid yourself. After a workout with Arnold and his friends I'm ready. Yes sir, World's is the place to be!

would sit and watch Arnold and Dave train. His Nikon was never out of reach. Art and his camera became a fixture at the gym. We hardly noticed him. Perhaps we even doubted he had any film in the camera. But what eventually resulted were the most amazing and realistic training photos ever seen. Pictures of Arnold rowing, benching, curling, and squatting, in which the weights were blurred by their motion; genuine perspiration stained the loose-fitting sweat tops; bars appeared to bend across the chest as they were bench-jetted upward; previously unrecorded facial expressions told the story of stress and pain and the single-minded, happy lunacy of hard-core training, all from the 35mm wide-angle lens of a humble, good-humored Santa Monica postman, who just happened to be the greatest muscle-recording camera artist alive.

One day when the gym was packed with

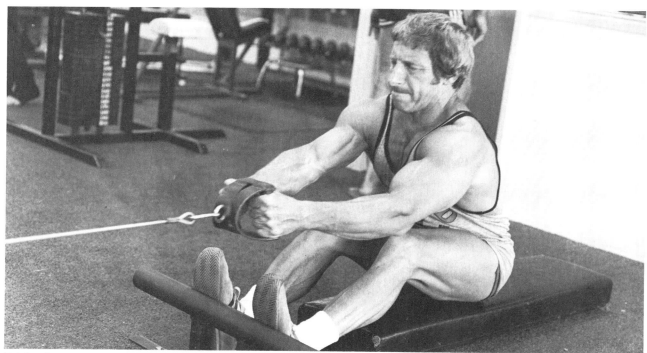

Eddie Giuliani trains daily at World Gym.

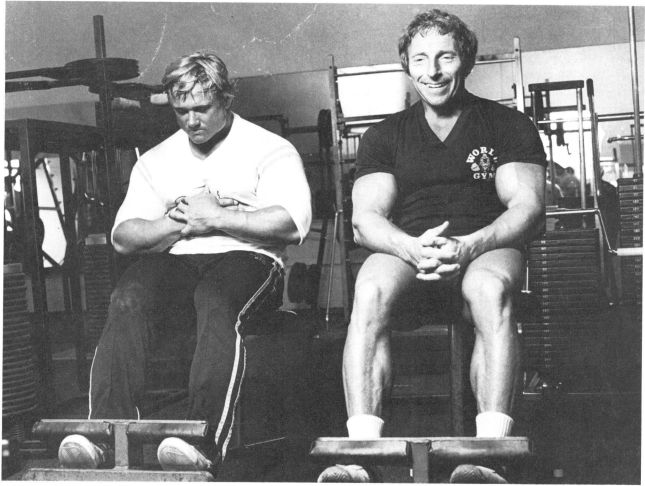

Eddie working out with one of the World Gym regulars, Tom Platz.

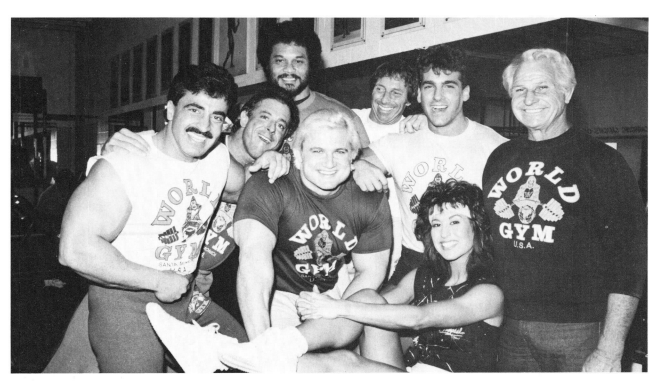
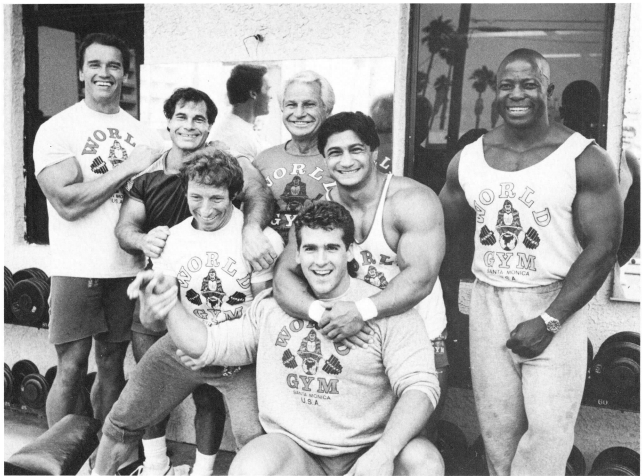

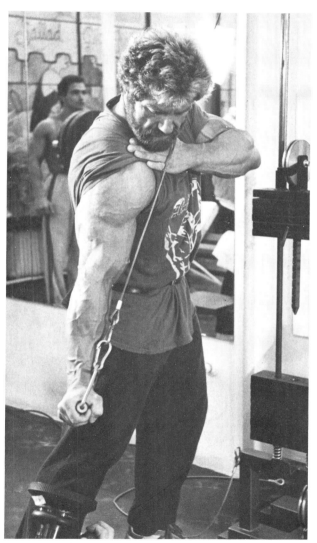

Jusup Wilcosz concentrates on developing his triceps.

WORLD WARFARE: THE FIVE-PART WORLD GYM MASTER PLAN

If there's one thing I've learned over the years, it is that there is more than one way to skin a cat! Of course I have my own ideas on training, but I have always resisted the temptation to be rigid in my thinking. Bodybuilding is after all a pretty loose type of activity. Rather than rules, we have guidelines. Instead of orders, we have suggestions.

World Gym trainers are the salt of the earth. There are literally hundreds of thousands of them. And they are the ones who have experimented with every conceivable training program, every diet, and every formula. These dedicated men and women, short or tall, fat or thin, champion or novice, young or not so young, have formulated the following five-part World Gym master plan.

- Priorities
- Physique
- Principles
- Preparation
- Personality

Start training today and put the World Gym trademark on your physique!

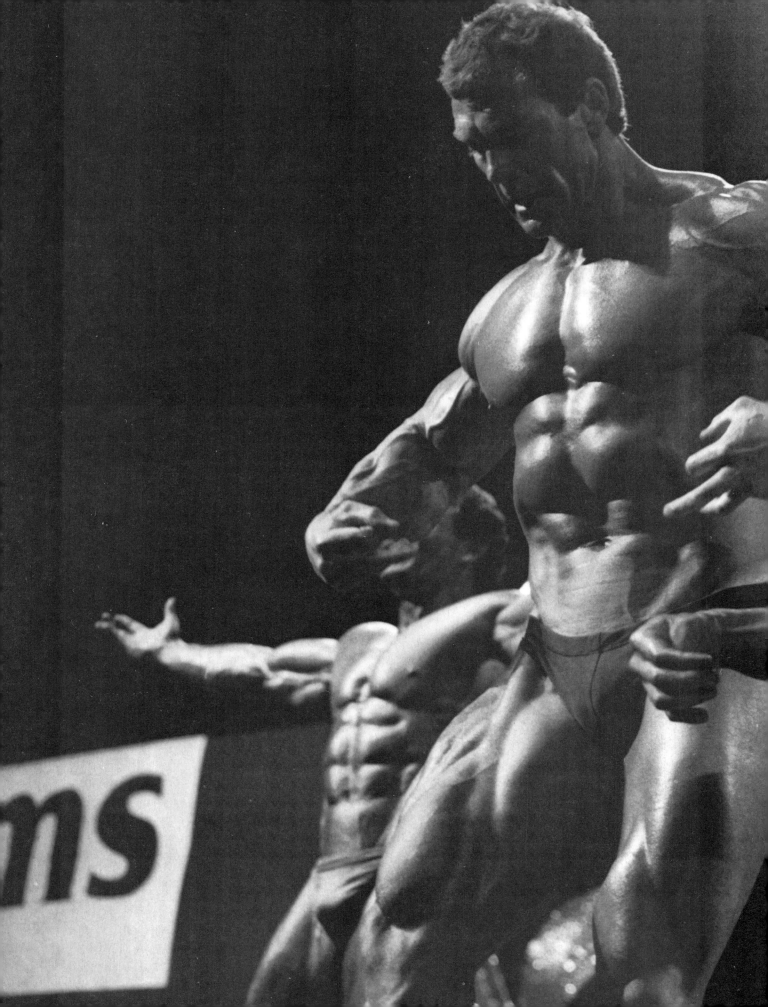

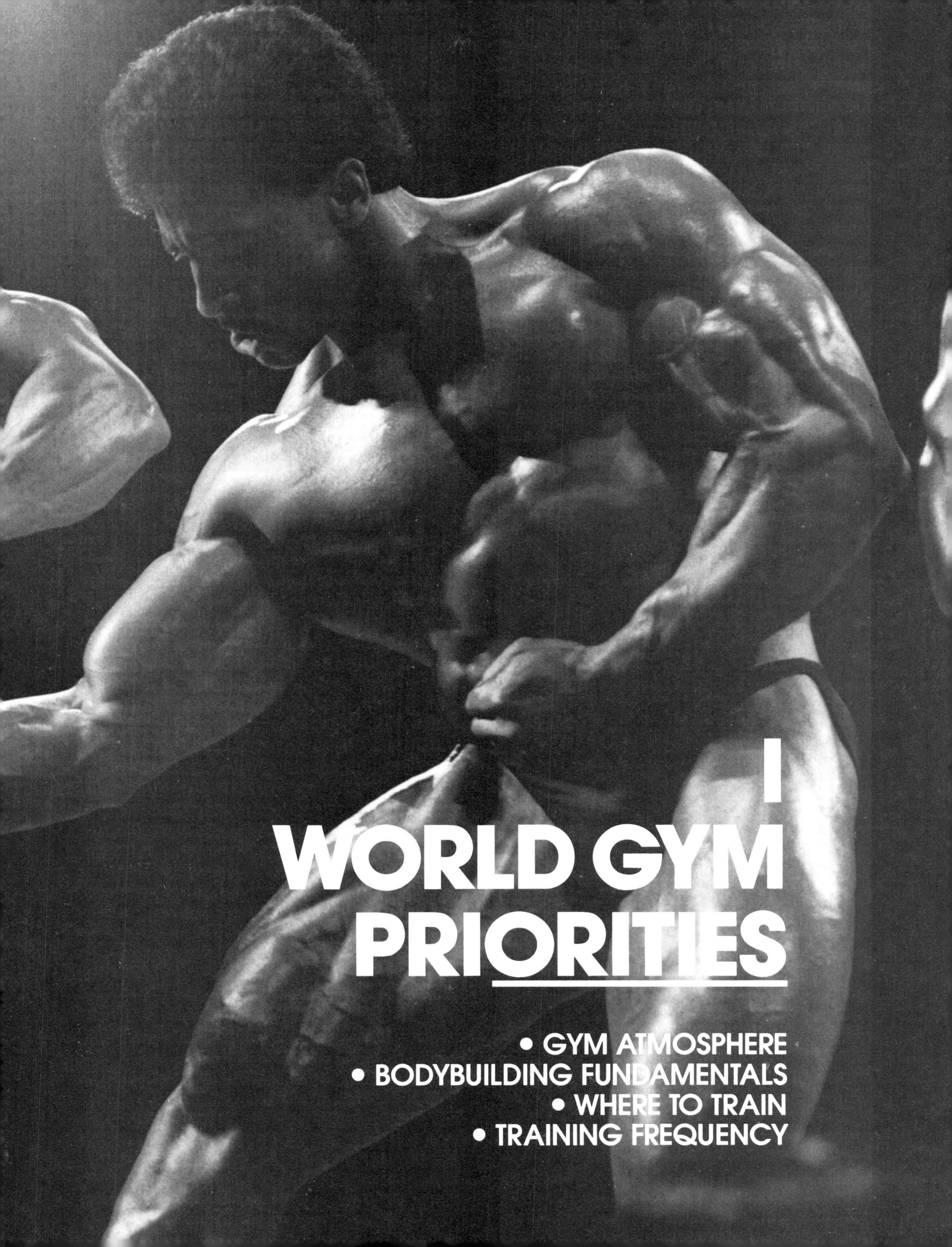

I
WORLD GYM
PRIORITIES

- GYM ATMOSPHERE
- BODYBUILDING FUNDAMENTALS
- WHERE TO TRAIN
- TRAINING FREQUENCY

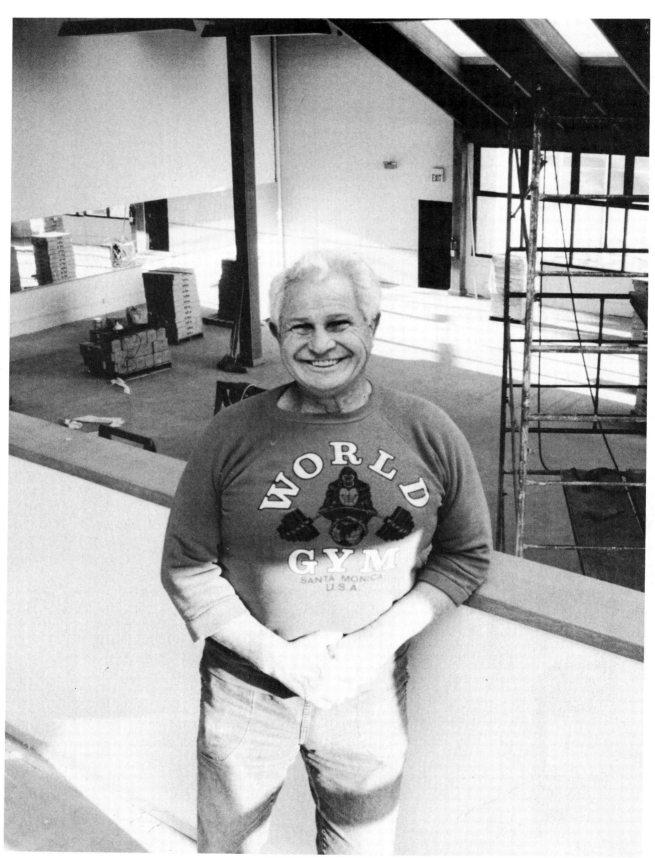

A proud Joe Gold shows off his new gym while under construction.

GYM ATMOSPHERE—THE RIGHT SETTING

When I first moved out of my native Los Angeles almost 40 years ago, it was because I didn't believe there was room for Vic Tanny and myself in the same town. Vic had several successful health studios underway, and I decided to follow in his footsteps. So my friend Chuck Krauser and I opened up a place in New Orleans called the Ajax Gym. We honestly believed that the Los Angeles area, with all of five gyms, was overloaded. Today there are hundreds of gyms in the Los Angeles area—all thriving—but being a perfectionist I always tried to make my training establishments different and better than the competition's.

Today my World Gym, at 812 Main Street in Venice, is considered the perfect environment for figure training, whether one is a star bodybuilder or simply a shape trainer in search of a steelworker's body.

Personally, I always enjoyed training *without* music (the sound of clanging plates and rhythmic breathing always seemed to me the right background for quality training). But that isn't to say that I wouldn't allow music if members preferred it. I've often joked that if my star member, Arnold Schwarzenegger, wanted music, I would have it piped in within the hour. Music can inspire you to train harder—if it's the right tempo. But you can't please everyone. Some like to train to

Roger Callard uses the quiet to concentrate on his upcoming lift.

15

classical music, while others like only hard rock.

Today it's not uncommon to see gyms with rows of machines set up like a supermarket. These places often seem more like factories than training establishments. Half the machines are not used. They just *look* impressive. I much prefer to have fewer machines and more space. If a machine is not used, I will toss it out. And the apparatus I have on the gym floor is serviced regularly. I find that by replacing cables when they're the least bit frayed, or by greasing the slightest squeak, I make the point that I want to keep the gym in the best possible condition. The members react to this by being careful with equipment and by respecting the facility in general. A gym is to be used, not abused, and if a member doesn't follow my exam-

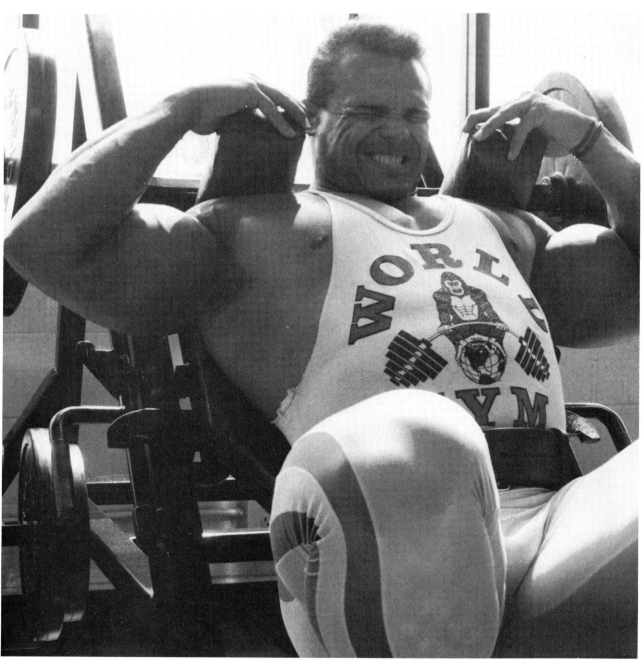

Brad Verret does some hacks.

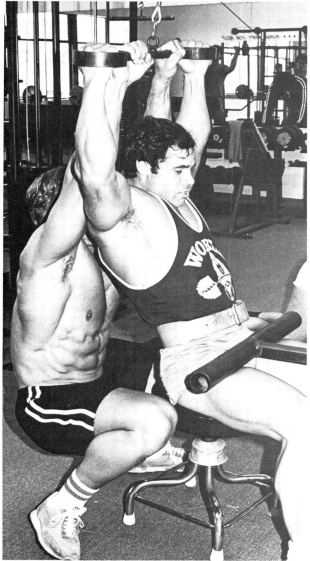

Arnold helps Franco on one of World Gym's personally designed machines.

ple, I will not hesitate to ask him to leave—for good.

John Balik, one of the most respected photographers in the business and publisher of *Iron Man* magazine, put it this way: "When you walk into World Gym, one of the first differences you notice between it and other gyms is that World's is an orderly place. There are no weights lying around, nobody carelessly dropping equipment; everything is in working order and in perfect repair." That's how I like it, and I intend to keep it that way.

Have you noticed that some gyms are like dungeons? There's no natural light at all. This is because many gyms are built in warehouse-type buildings. Industrial space is cheaper to rent than Class A commercial. And basements are the cheapest of all. One visit to World's in Venice will give you an idea of what a complete bodybuilding environment is all about. We have space, high ceilings, skylights, and enormous windows that let in just the right amount of daylight. You feel inspired to train to the max, and that's what it's all about.

I am fussy over the apparatus I have in my gyms. Years ago, there just wasn't any good stuff around. If we wanted to do inclines, we just propped a flat bench up on a box so that it was set at an angle. Pretty soon, as an aspiring bodybuilder aware of the importance of "angle training," I got a doctor friend of mine to show me how to use a welding torch. From then on, by trial and error, I created what many believe to be the most result-producing apparatus available anywhere. But it didn't happen overnight. My backyard was full of benches and pulley and lat machines that weren't quite perfect. To get to where my machines are today took me a lifetime of mistakes and miscalculations. Typically, I would get one part of a machine perfect, but in so doing it would affect some other area. When I first invented the adjustable incline bench it worked great, but the lower the angle the more likely you were to slip off the seat pad. We used to put our feet up on a dumbbell rack to hold ourselves in position. One day, in the middle of a set, another gym member wanted to use the dumbbells right where my feet were resting. I still remember his whispered curse as he was forced to wait for me to finish my set. That night I invented a seat pad with an easily adjustable angle. We never had to put our feet up on the dumbbell rack again.

People often ask me why Arnold Schwarzenegger always trains at my gym. It is obvious that he could train at the most private and exclusive gyms in Los

Angeles. I have known Arnold for over 20 years now and I've never asked him why he likes World Gym best. I guess it's simply that Arnold still prefers to train like the champions, and with the champions. His workouts are not so grueling as in his Olympia-winning years, but he still likes to train on heavy-duty apparatus and with free weights—and he's not averse to hard work, especially when a film role is coming up in which he has to be in tip-top condition. Arnold also knows that when he's in the company of other World Gym members he will not be bugged for advice or plagued for autographs. When he's training, his privacy is respected; and if by chance some undesirable did start to bug him, I would waste no time in acting as the great protector.

Not only did I design my gym in Venice but I supervised every part of its construction, from the first to the last brick. I put everything into the venture, and I'm proud of the achievement, but I'm never totally satisfied. A gym has to grow and change, and with that in mind I'm always looking for ways to improve.

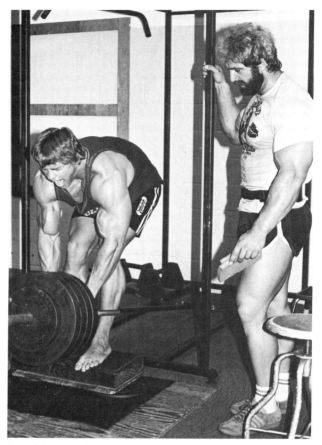

Arnold trains his back as Jusup looks on.

BODYBUILDING FUNDAMENTALS— STARTING RIGHT

It's like anything else. Getting into body-building is easy. If you know how!

There's no doubt in my mind that progressive-resistance exercise (weight training) is extremely worthwhile. Barbells and dumbbells are *tools* that can work a magic you will not find elsewhere. If used with care and intelligence you can shape, build, or reduce your body at will. Use them as a sculptor does his hammer and chisel. Eat according to your goals, more if you want to gain mass, less if you want to trim down. Always eat natural, wholesome foods.

STARTING OUT

Before beginning any type of formal exercise or undergoing a change in your eating habits, see your doctor and explain what you are going to do. Chances are he'll be delighted you're thinking about regular exercise, but if you are over 40, a heavy smoker, or if there is a history of heart, organ, or circulatory problems, he will probably have you undergo a simple stress test to make sure that you can handle a vigorous exercise program. Don't worry— it's not painful, and after your doctor gives you the all-clear, you will be that much more confident in your aspirations to build the perfect body.

THE TOOLS OF THE TRADE

I have always used basic barbells, dumbbells, and weight-loaded machines in my training, and despite the modern trend toward gimmicky exercise apparatus that comes in all shapes and sizes, I still firmly believe that the free-weight system is the best game in town.

The beauty of free weights is that you can use them effectively whether you are weak or strong, short or tall, young or not so young. Free-weight disks come in all sizes (from $1\frac{1}{4}$ pounds to 100 pounds), and you can tailor a particular barbell or dumbbell set to your strength level. There need be no strain or red-faced huffing and puffing; no injuries and no overwork. The modern disk-loading barbell can be made right for you in every exercise you do, and in just a matter of seconds.

THE ROUTINE

A normal workout is made up of a variety of exercises that work the different muscles of the body. All the muscles should be trained two to four times a week, depending on your goals. A well-balanced routine involves performing about eight to fifteen movements. There are actually thousands of different weight-training exercises for every part of the body, but my more than 50 years of experience has shown me that some exercises are more effective than others. It is these exercises that I am advocating.

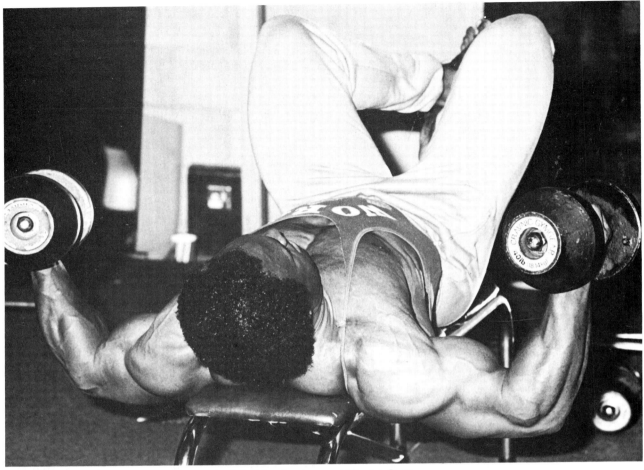

Three-time Mr. Olympia Lee Haney builds his physique at World Gym.

MEN AND WOMEN

The question often comes up: should men and women train in the same way? Is there a difference between the sexes when it comes to bodybuilding exercises? Well, both men and women have the same muscles, and the short answer is that both should train identically. There are, however, physical characteristics that are seen more on women than on men, and vice versa. Women tend to have wider hips, narrower shoulders, and smaller joints than men. Men often possess more muscular thighs and glutes and less overall body fat. But these are only generalizations. We all know women with broad shoulders and big bones; and many have naturally low body-fat levels. And men with wide hips, fatty thighs, and narrow shoulders are not exactly uncommon.

Whereas training has to be tailored to our individual requirements, it is too much of a generalization to divide the schedules automatically between men and women because of some stereotype we may have formulated.

When it comes to building muscle it is true that men can build more muscle and at a faster rate than women. They tend to be stronger in the arms, shoulders, chest, and upper back. But hold on—women are frequently stronger than men in leg, hip, and lower-back movements. This makes for very compatible workout partners. Although the men will invariably use more weight, a woman often trains for longer periods, with more intensity, and frequently with a perfect exercise style. Each sex teaches the other something worthwhile: the man encourages the use of heavier weights, while the woman influences the man to train longer, with more intensity, and with better form.

SETS AND REPS

A repetition, or "rep" as it is known among bodybuilders, is one count of an exercise. One floor dip, for example, is one rep. Two squats are two reps, and so on. When you perform several nonstop reps of a particular exercise before putting the weight down for a breather, that is known as a set. After a minute or so you may again pick up the weight and perform more reps before again taking a short rest. A single series of 10 squats, for example, would be known as one set of 10 reps. When this is written it appears like this: Squats—1 × 10. Should you perform, say, three sets of barbell curls with 12 reps in each set, this would appear as: Barbell Curl—3 × 12.

WHAT TO WEAR

The gym can be quite a fashionable place, although its main function is to help you build health, strength, physique, and vitality. It is also a friendly place, although I hasten to add that a good, functional gym should never be known as a pickup joint.

Your main concerns in training apparel should be warmth and comfort. You can look attractive while you train, but make sure you're comfortable. Warm muscles function better and pump easier. A good, full-length track suit is hard to beat, although many trainers prefer to wear skin-tight garments that highlight the legs and glutes to the max. In cold weather do not hesitate to wear several layers of loose clothing. Better to be too hot than too cold, and as you warm up you can always shed a layer or two.

Never train barefoot or with thong sandals. You could stub your toe or even drop a weight, and end your training for the day—or even the month.

Always wear shoes. Running shoes with a built-in support are best. Couple these with thick woolen socks that allow the feet to breathe while absorbing sweat.

In really hot temperatures, shorts and a

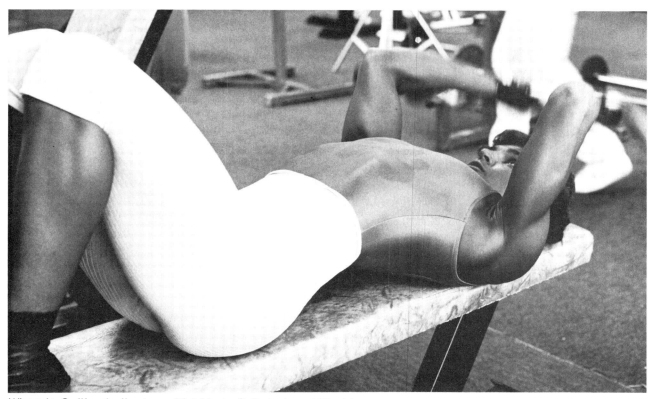

When in California the beautiful Marjo Selin trains at World.

tank top may be ideal. Seeing your muscles in action while you force out the reps can do wonders for your pump!

SAFETY IN TRAINING

There are not many sports that are safer than weight training, but you should still observe a few basic rules. First and fore-

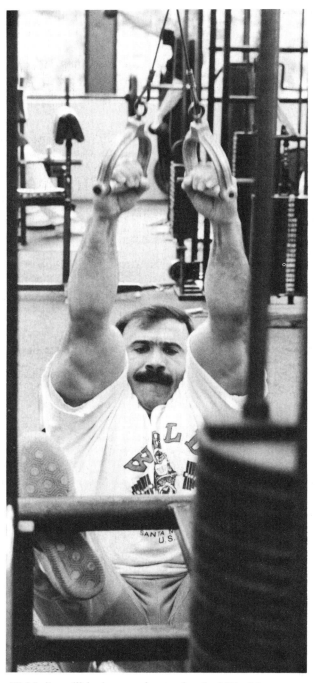

Ali Malla will train no where else but World.

most you should never randomly pick up a heavy weight to "see if you can lift it." This is inviting trouble in the form of a muscle tear or strain. More lower backs have been "put out" by ego-induced sloppy lifting than any other reason.

Never train alone on heavy movements such as the bench press or squat, where if you fail to lift the bar you are trapped in an awkward position. I can't count the number of times someone training without spotters in my gym has called out for help because he had become caught under a heavy weight. I dread to think what would happen if I weren't around to help.

If you're an experienced bodybuilder, you may not think this applies to you. It does. Every experienced weight trainer I've ever known has come up against injury of some kind, and in virtually every case it could have been avoided. Don't get the wrong idea—bodybuilding *is* a safe sport, probably the safest, but you still have to use good old-fashioned common sense. The following is a list of the most common ways you can injure yourself. In my 50-odd years of association with bodybuilding I have repeatedly witnessed gym members doing all of the following:

- Dropping weights on their feet.
- Letting their egos run wild and trying to lift a stray barbell or dumbbell that is far too heavy.
- Handing off a bar incorrectly after bench-pressing and having it drop onto their chests.
- Loading and unloading heavy barbells without consideration for what can happen to a barbell that is much heavier on one side than the other.
- Failure to warm up with a light to moderate weight before going to the limit on a particular set.
- Adopting sloppy exercise habits of bouncing and heaving the weights rather than keeping total control of the resistance.

Did you hear about the physique star who let one weak moment ruin his career

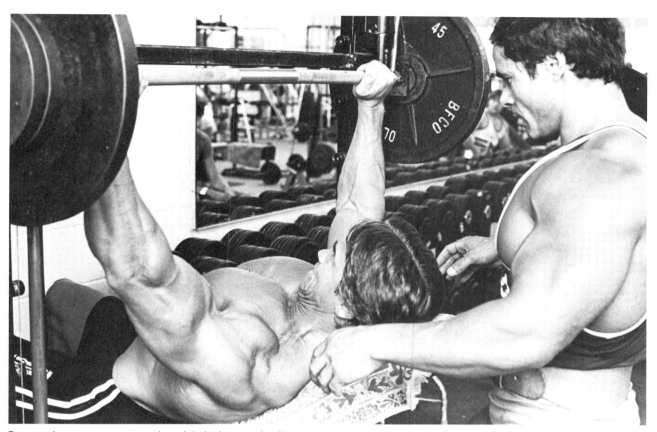

Franco keeps an eye on Arnold during an incline press.

in bodybuilding? This scene took place at a North American training establishment.

The fellow in question, who incidentally possesses among the biggest muscular arms in the sport, 21¾", was being photographed at one end of the gym. Special photo floodlights surrounded him. He was completely oiled up to highlight his muscles. The camera was firing repeatedly, capturing pose after pose. . . .

"You're just a *pretty* boy," shouted one of the gym's bearded powerlifting fraternity, obviously jealous of our subject's proportions. "You don't have any *real* strength. What good are all those muscles without *real* strength?" A few snickers followed as if to give credence to the remarks.

Well, that did it. The posing stopped, and our subject ran down to where the abusive powerlifter was training. An Olympic bar loaded to 435 pounds was cradled on the bench. The physique man, still oiled up, plonked himself down on his back, determined to show the heckler just

how strong his "pretty" muscles were. He hurriedly lifted the weight from the racks, determined to rep-out a set of eight strict reps—and then it happened. No sooner had he lifted the bar from the supports than his oil-covered hands slipped outward, collar to collar—and the weight came tumbling down. Our ego-activated physiqueman sustained a torn pectoral muscle and a ripped biceps. He will never compete successfuly as a bodybuilder again.

Bob Kennedy, publisher of *MuscleMag International*, told me of an incident that happened two years ago when he met his former art college pal Gino Edwards at MuscleMag's Muscle Store in Brampton, Canada. After some preliminary catch-up conversation, Bob pointed to a 120-pound dumbbell on the floor. "Remember the days when we could press that overhead one-handed with ease?" Bob laughed. Forgetting the 25-year lapse in time, Gino accepted Bob's joking remark as a personal challenge. He took a couple of deep breaths, bent over the dumbbell, and without any warm-up whatsoever hoisted it to his shoulder and cheat-pressed it for four reps. That little act of foolishness earned a round of applause from Bob and a somewhat impressed customer who just happened to be around. It also earned Gino a torn trapezius and a pinched nerve condition that has to this day robbed his right arm of 80 percent of its function!

When you are bench-pressing always make sure you hand off the weight safely. If you are replacing the barbell onto a rack, make absolutely certain you drop the bar into *both* cradles. Sometimes, after a particularly strenuous set, one is tempted to dump off the weight carelessly, trusting that the bar will hit the cradles correctly.

Risky business, indeed. Missing your target can mean the end of your face. Take care!

The same thing applies to your use of training partners. Make sure your spotter has a firm grip on the bar before you let go. It is vital that you *never* release your grip until the bar is no longer directly over your head.

Exercising in cold conditions makes muscle tears and strains more likely. If the temperature is on the cool side, cover up with several layers of loose clothing. Far better that your muscles are too warm than too cold. A warm muscle will respond better to exercise. It is stronger and will pump up more efficiently. Some people like to wear only a tank top while training. They reason that when they can see the

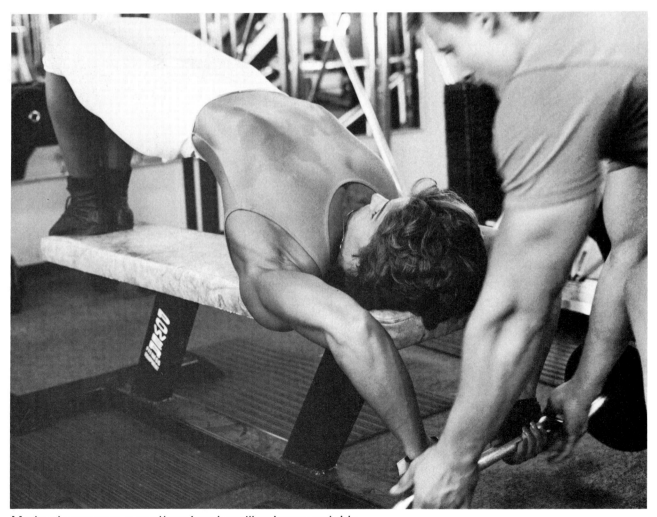

Marjo always uses a spotter when handling heavy weights.

muscle working, they get a better pump. This is fine, but never shed a long-sleeved garment for a short-sleeved one unless you are sure the gym temperature is warm enough to nurture a pump. My original World Gym in Venice had an outdoor training deck that gave gym members the option of training outside if they wished. This was so successful that I have two outdoor training areas in my new World Gym.

California weather being what it is, more than 300 sunny days every year, these outdoor decks make perfect sense, but I would be the last person to recommend that anyone train outdoors if the weather is less than warm and balmy.

You must do everything reasonable to avoid injury. This includes warming up thoroughly for every exercise. Beginners will need only one warm-up set, but as you become more advanced you may find you need two or three sets to get your muscles humming. The pro bodybuilders who train at my gym often use the pyramid style of training in order to warm up their muscles progressively; that is to say, weights are added every set until the last two or three sets are done with resistance at or near the limit. Advanced bodybuilders use pyramiding in heavy exercises such as squats and bench presses.

If you've been around gyms for a while, you will have seen what happens when you load or unload a supported barbell more on one side than the other. It flips! And big damage can be done. As a result of this careless maneuver the bar can swing into the air and the weights crash to the floor. It's amazing how many people fail to use common sense when loading or unloading a supported barbell, because this mistake occurs again and again.

Always use collars when training, especially on overhead lifts. Weights have a way of working over to one side, and this occurs even more frequently if you are using heavy poundage in loose exercise style. I can't count the times I have seen inexperienced people attempting to lift a heavy weight overhead, only to have the

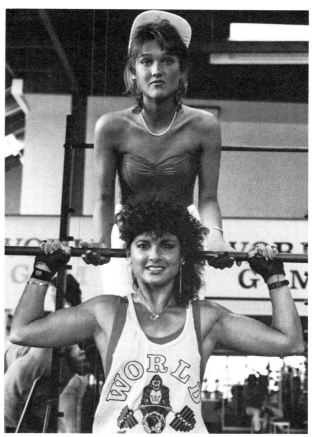

Some of the women of World.

weights on one side of the bar slide off, followed quickly by those from the other side. It's a double crash that tends to annoy us gym owners, especially if we have just installed new carpets. And while I'm on the subject of carpets, I'll let you in on a pet peeve of mine. I do not like to see any member of my World Gym dragging a bench across the gym floor. If you want to move a piece of equipment, that's fine, but you had better lift it clear off the floor. Dragging equipment is not acceptable to me. It marks, scratches, and tears expensive flooring or carpets. I have a motto on the subject, and heaven help you if I have to shout it at you: "If you can't lift it, don't move it!"

Throughout this book I explain the proper way to perform the various exercises. Whereas there is room for variation in some movements, it is important that the basic body positions be adhered to. The body must be set correctly to lift,

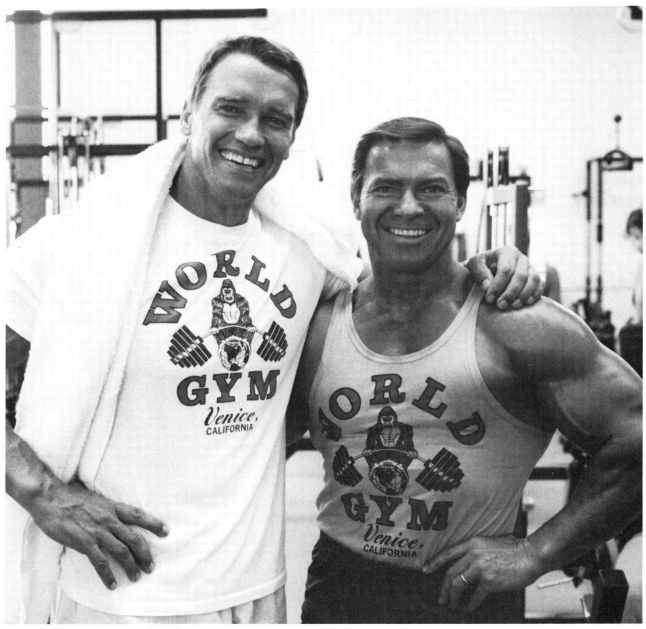

Arnold and the ageless Larry Scott.

whether it be your arms, chest, legs, or back that does the work. There must be a functional biomechanical correctness to each exercise position. Deviating from this proper biomechanical position, especially when using heavy weights, can leave you open to injury. For example, squatters and deadlifters should always strive to keep their backs flat. Never turn your head to one side while squatting. When bench-pressing, never bounce the weight on your chest. A cracked sternum can result from this habit.

When taking a loaded barbell from a rack (for squats or behind-neck presses), make sure you don't lift it up until you're solidly under the weight, knees bent, back flat, head up. The same position also applies to standing calf raises when you first increase the resistance before the first heel-raise repetition.

Don't neglect to use a good leather weight-lifting belt for your heavy exercises. A belt is necessary for movements such as rows, deadlifts, squats, and standing presses. It gives you support and confidence, and once you learn how to *use* a belt to your advantage, you'll find it enables you to use heavier weights, which invariably translates to bigger muscles. And that is what you want, isn't it? A belt supports the entire midsection. It protects the lower back and holds in the waist area. Frank Zane wears his belt the *wrong* way round when squatting, so that the wide area covers his waistline. "This holds my abdominals intact," he says. "The heavy pushing involved in squats can distend the waistline area, so I minimize the possiblility by wearing my lifting belt the wrong way round. It works!"

Finally, don't litter the floor with loose disks, odd barbells, dumbbells, collars, and sleeves. Sooner or later you'll stub your toe, trip over a weight, or step on a loose bar and land on your back. You don't put only yourself in danger; you could be risking injury to others. Here's a playback of what happened in one gym recently. After a set of heavy dumbbell presses, a bodybuilder returned the weights to the racks so carelessly that he caught his finger, cutting it badly. He reacted by veering around sharply and hitting another member who was carrying a barbell to a Scott bench. He in turn twisted away, hurting his back and dropping his barbell on the foot of a woman doing bench presses, who herself was so shocked (and pained) that she dropped the weight on her clavicle. Net result of the carelessness: one severely cut thumb, a twisted vertebra, a bruised toe, and a cracked collar bone. Yes, safety rules are important.

WHERE TO TRAIN

Basically, you have two choices: Either you train in a home gym or at a commercial gym such as World's. Both have advantages.

HOME GYM TRAINING

The greatest plus in favor of training at home is that you can train at any time. Your home is always there, ready for use.

Should the weather be bad, especially if the nearest commercial gym is far away, you do not have the additional hassle of having to make the time-consuming, often arduous trip to and from the establishment.

Addtionally, when you train at home you never have to wait in line to use certain pieces of equipment, nor do you have to deal socially with people you may not like. You can play your own kind of music on the radio—or have no music at all.

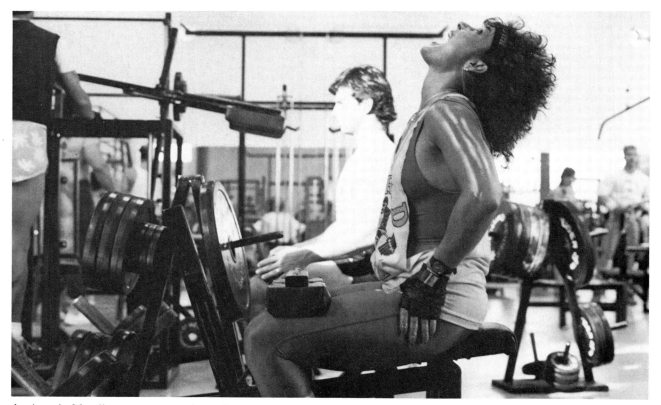

Andrea LeMantia squeezes out another rep on the seated calf machine.

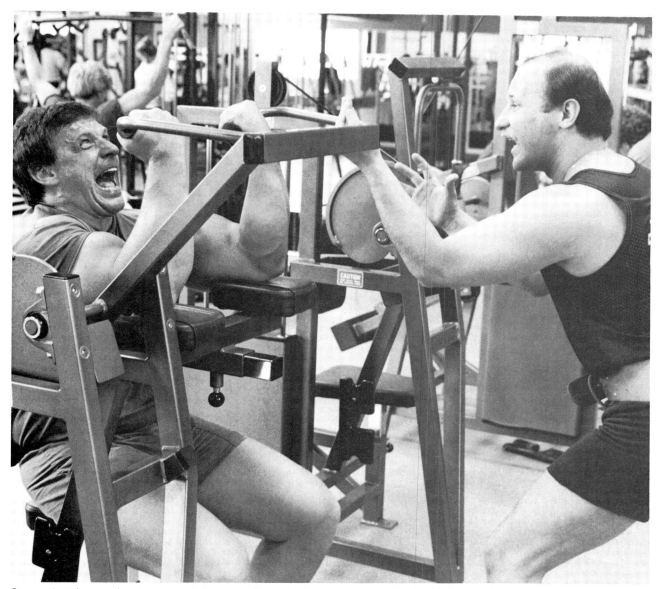

One advantage of a commercial gym is the variety of equipment on which to train.

COMMERCIAL GYM TRAINING

Every advanced bodybuilder trains extensively at commerical gyms. Multi-Mr. Olympia Lee Haney spent more than $30,000 equipping his home gym but admits that just before Olympia time he has to train in a commercial establishment to reach peak condition.

You always have a greater selection of equipment at a commerical gym. There is more competition. When you train in the company of others, you gain faster, especially if they are stronger and more physically advanced. You will invariably work harder and faster and not be tempted to read or watch TV between sets as so many home-gym trainers do.

TRAINING FREQUENCY—
HOW OFTEN IS BEST?

How often you train depends on several factors, the most important being your availability. Obviously, if you are going to school and working at a job, you will not be able to train as often as you might wish. Some people have two jobs; others have family obligations they don't want to neglect. Training frequency is also affected by your energy level, recuperative ability, and overall condition.

Not so long ago most trainers exercised the whole body three times a week. This usually translated to Monday, Wednesday, and Friday training, leaving a full day's rest between workouts and the weekend entirely free. This method is still popular and certainly presents a workable plan. But it often leads to excessively long workouts that can take several hours to complete, assuming of course that you have the inspiration and energy to see a marathon workout through to the end.

Physiologists have concluded that it takes a muscle something in excess of 48 hours to fully recuperate, and that blitzing the same muscle again before it has fully recovered serves no practical purpose. As a result, many bodybuilders began experimenting with training frequency, especially in relation to dividing workouts into different parts.

One common practice is to divide your routine into two approximately equal halves. Perform the first half on day one and the second half on day two. On day three you rest. The next workout (day four), you perform the first half of your routine again, and then on day five you train on the second half. Day six is a rest day. This simple frequency plan works well for most bodybuilders. Here are some variations:

THE THREE-DAY-ON, ONE-DAY-OFF ROUTINE

Divide your routine into three fairly equal parts. Perform the first part on day one, the second part on day two, and the third part on day three. Day four is your rest day, after which you start the cycle again. This method works each body part twice weekly.

Day One
Legs, glutes, triceps
Day Two
Chest, biceps, forearms
Day Three
Shoulders, back, traps, abs

EVERY OTHER DAY SPLIT

More and more bodybuilders are turning to this method of training, which was popularized by none other than Mike Mentzer. It is usually a satisfactory "growing" method, especially if used in conjunction with high-intensity workouts. It's a super way to build size and power in the off-season.

Divide your routine into two equal

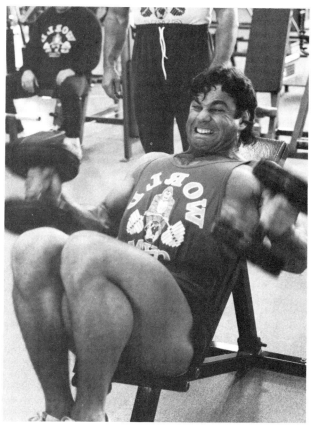

Jon-Jon Park does some seated hammer curls for full development of the biceps.

ideal training frequency for yourself. But always keep in mind that a muscle group should not be worked excessively more than three times a week, nor less than one and a half times a week (preferably two).

Some bodybuilders like to divide their routine into upper-body and lower-body sections. Accordingly, one day they train their chest, back, delts, and arms, and devote the next workout to the thighs, glutes, hamstrings, and calves. Still another variation is to divide a routine into all "pushing" exercises and all "pulling" exercises. Typical pushing exercises would be standing, seated, and lying presses and triceps movements; "pulling" exercises include thigh curls, deadlifts, upright and bent-over rowing, lat pulldowns, seated pulley rows, and chins.

halves. Perform the first half on day one. Day two is a rest day. Then perform the second half of your workout on day three and take day four off. Now you are ready to start the cycle again. You never train two days in a row. The only problem with this routine is that it doesn't fit in with the normal work week. There will be times when you will have to train on Sundays. This may not fit in with your gym's hours, or with your family commitments.

THE TWO-DAYS-ON, ONE-DAY-OFF ROUTINE

Divide your workout program into two equal halves. Perform the first half on day one, the second half the next day, and rest up on the third day. Then repeat the cycle. This frequency does not give you free weekends; if that's not a problem, it can be an ideal system for gaining size and strength.

With a little ingenuity you can plan an

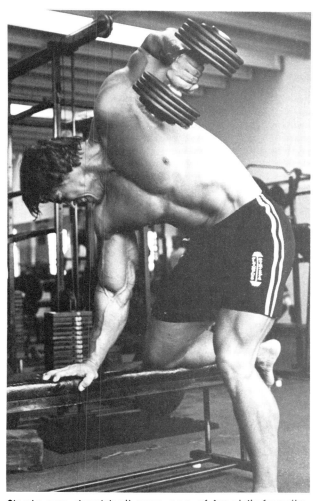

Single-arm dumbbell rows, one of Arnold's favorite exercises for his back.

Also remember that as a competition approaches, it is often a good idea to increase training frequency from twice weekly to three times weekly. This invites burnout from overtiredness and underrecuperation, so four to six weeks of this advanced frequency is usually all you can take without losing strength and mass.

Advanced trainers, especially the pro bodybuilders, make use of the fact that they can train at any time by splitting their workout routines a second time so that they can work out twice a day. A few even train three times a day, but these can be counted on the fingers of one hand.

It's not unusual, however, for a pro bodybuilder to train thighs in the morning and then return in the evening to train abs and calves. Several bodybuilders I know train one body part in one gym and then go for a little lunch, lie on the beach, and proceed to another gym to train a second body part. Nice work if you can get it!

The most important thing about choosing your workout frequency is recuperation. It's no good training a body part

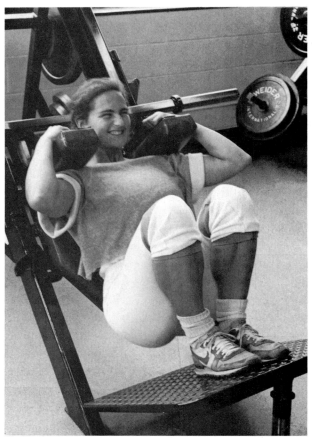

Hacks are essential for fully developed quads as demonstrated by Shawn Stouffer.

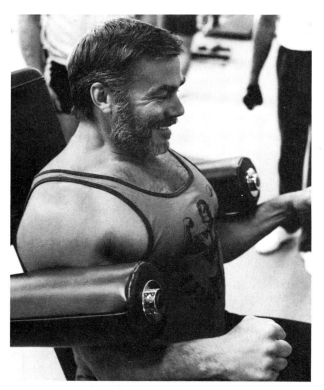

Sven Ole Thorsen does a machine lat raise.

three or four times a week if you can't fully recuperate from the muscle stimulation. Overtrain and you will drag your body into a sticking point, or you may even cause gains to be lost.

It is vital when changing training frequency to take it easy the first few workouts. Don't push yourself excessively at this early stage. You must break into your new mode of training quietly, holding back on your enthusiasm for the first few workouts or until your body has adjusted to the new training rhythm. Then you can go to two on to the higher sets with increased intensity. But always be aware of your recuperative levels.

BREATHING PATTERNS

Naturally we have to breathe during our exercises, but many beginners are confused about when and how they should

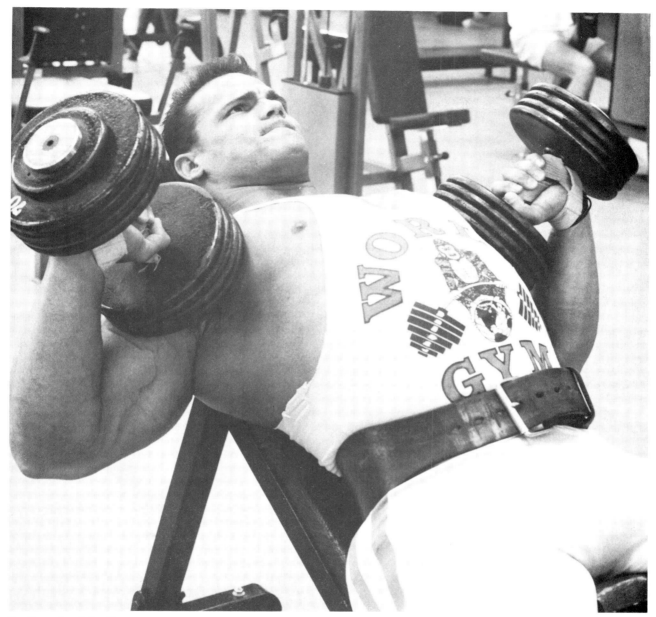

For the chest, incline presses.

breathe. In most cases, you inhale and exhale once for every repetition. The usual pattern is to breathe in during the easiest part of the exercise (before starting the rep) and breathe out as you complete the hardest part. Use your mouth. The nose channels are too small to inhale adequate oxygen during vigorous exercise. You should gulp in air, then exhale it under control through pursed lips. Some body-builders sound like steam engines in the middle of a heavy set. Try to keep some control because excessive noise can interfere with the concentration of others.

In exercises such as calf raises, abdominal lifts, lat rows, and trap shrugs you may find that you only need to breathe in every two or three reps. Find out which tempo suits training and adapt accordingly. Try not to hold your breath during heavy exercises such as overhead or bench presses. You could black out from a temporary lack of oxygen (the valsalva effect) and drop the weight, causing injury.

REST, SLEEP, AND RECUPERATION

When you exercise a muscle vigorously, the muscle fiber breaks down and requires a period of rest to recuperate. That is why you should never train the same muscle group heavily two days in a row if you are hoping to build it to a larger size. Those of you who are trying to add mass should aim to get at least eight hours of sleep nightly. Even more may be recommended.

Some pro bodybuilders in competition training take a half hour afternoon nap to restore their energy and freshness. I realize that this custom, while acceptable at siesta time in Mexico or Spain, may or may not be practical for the average working man or woman in today's fast-paced society.

I should point out that those trying to gain weight will find their task easier if they are employed as office or desk workers rather than road laborers or manual workers.

Peace of mind is also vital. Avoid emotionally draining situations, arguments, and frustrating or volatile circumstances, if at all possible.

RECORD KEEPING

Recording your exercises, poundage used, and the number of sets and reps can be helpful. Right now you may not be inclined to do this, but, believe me, in a few years when you look back on the statistics of today's workouts you will get a kick out of contrasting the various data. But it's more than that: keeping count of what you do each workout can help you with your progression. If you want to make progress,

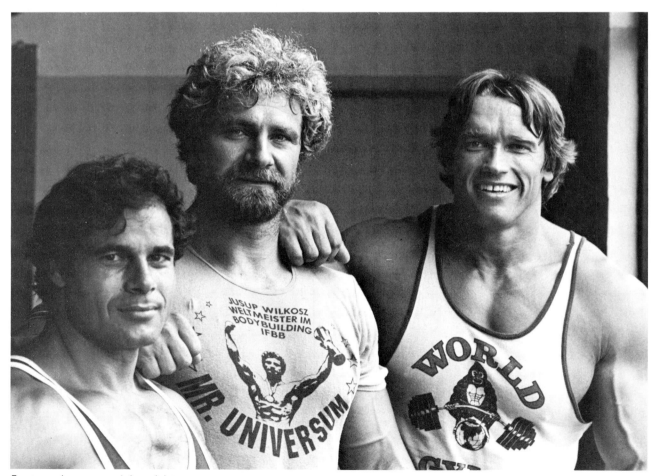

Franco, Jusup, and Arnold.

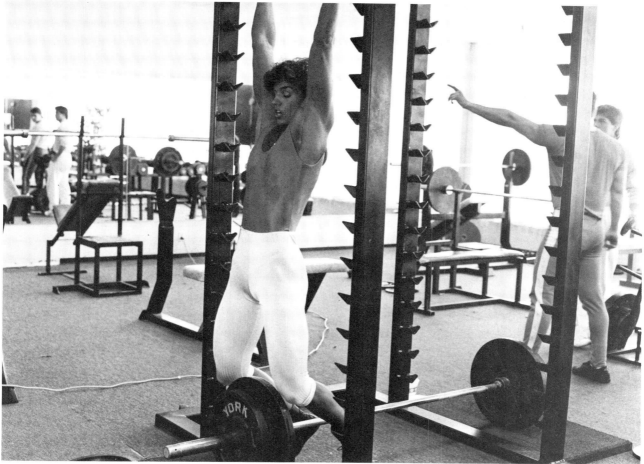

Marjo Selin stretching her back after a set of deadlifts.

you have to push yourself to do more while not allowing your workouts to become excessively drawn out. A record book will help make your tasks easier. In addition, you can record your measurements, weight, and even your food intake.

You seldom notice a great deal of advancement in the poundages you use from day to day or week to week, but with a training log, you can flick a page and be able to check back six months or a year. And you'll get a heck of a boost in your training when you realize what great progress you're making.

GENETICS

Bodybuilding genetics are those intangibles that are handed down in your genes, courtesy of your forefathers. Some of us

are born healthy and strong, while others get a somewhat poorer start. The truth is that while just about anyone can benefit from regular bodybuilding exercise, only a few of us can go all the way to the top of the championship ladder. When all is said and done, there can only be one Mr. and Ms. Olympia each year. "Choosing the right parents is the surest way to body-building success," says Arnold Schwarzenegger, but he cautions that there are dozens of other variables to the success formula—hard work, consistency, and goal-setting being just three.

One barometer of your ability to do well in this sport is skeletal size and muscle-cell counts. Good testosterone levels are also vital for men. It's not easy to determine if you have the type of body that is championship material. Many skinny

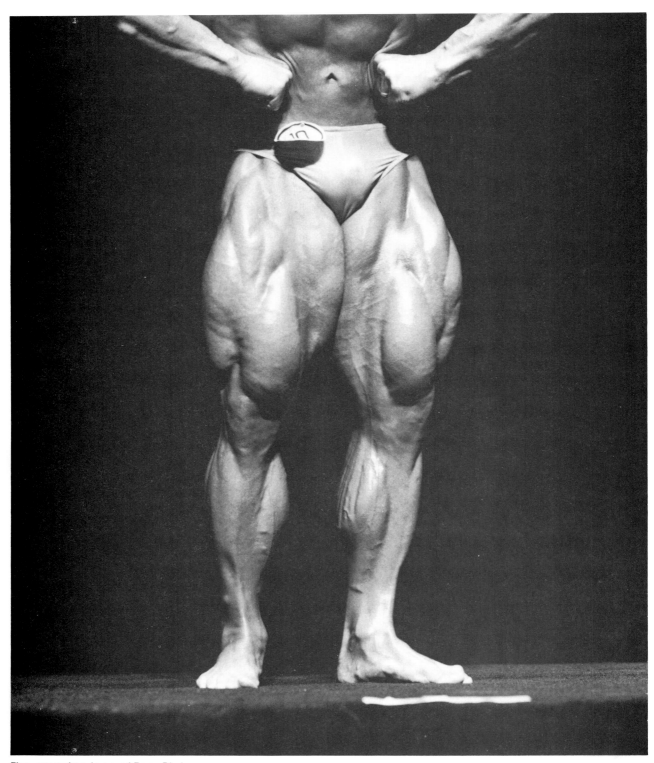

The amazing legs of Tom Platz.

bodybuilders, such as Danny Padilla and Samir Bannout, have gained enough quality mass to win international titles. The same goes for those who were overweight. Tom Platz and Juliette Bergman are two such people. But skinny or fat each of these individuals was blessed with muscle cells of high integrity, good skeletal structures, and ideal muscle insertions, not to mention a predisposition for mental fortitude and an unharnessed ambition to succeed and be recognized.

CONSISTENCY

What was it Thomas Edison said? "Success is 10 percent inspiration and 90 percent perspiration." Well, whatever the percentages involved, it is an indisputable fact that bodybuilding requires perseverance. This is not a part-time sport in which an on-and-off trainer succeeds. Those bodybuilders who find themselves torn between a show biz career and competition success invariably have to sacrifice one for the other.

You have to be consistent in your workouts. Naturally, if you are sick with the flu or have a severe headache, you should not work out, nor should you train if you are excessively tired. But learn to differentiate between genuine tiredness and laziness. The latter should *never* keep you away from the gym.

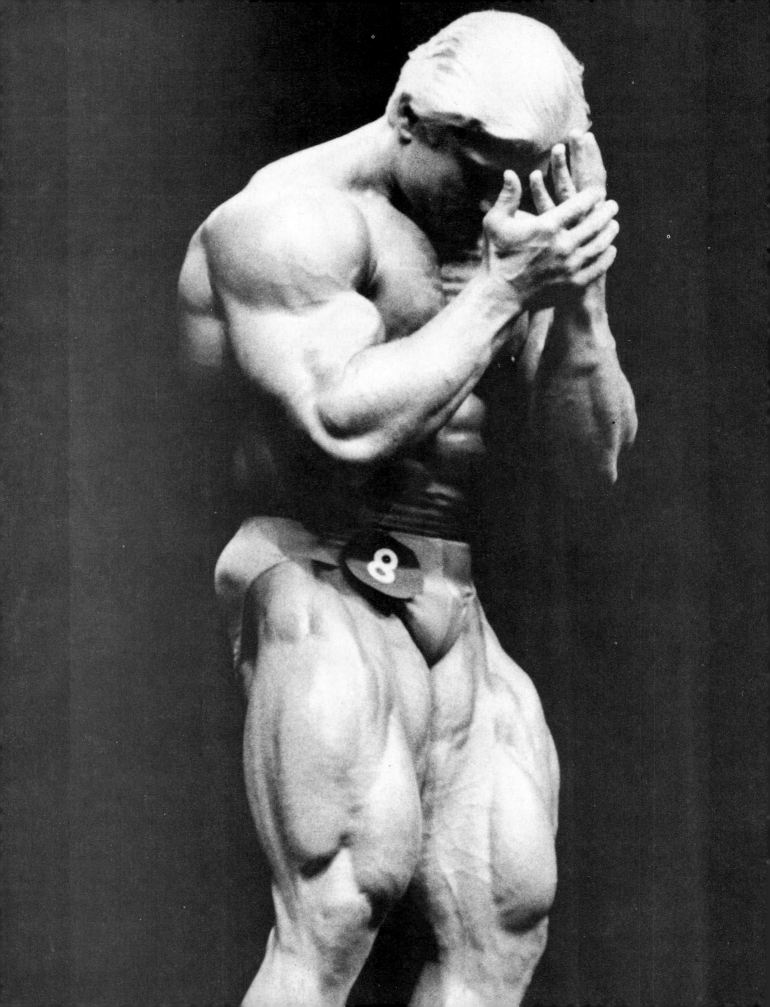

II
WORLD GYM PHYSIQUE

- MIND OVER MATTER
- YOUR FIRST ROUTINE
- SHAPE TRAINING
- HARDCORE TRAINING STRATEGIES
- EMPIRICAL TRAINING
- FEEDER WORKOUTS
- WORLD GYM SUPERSTARS

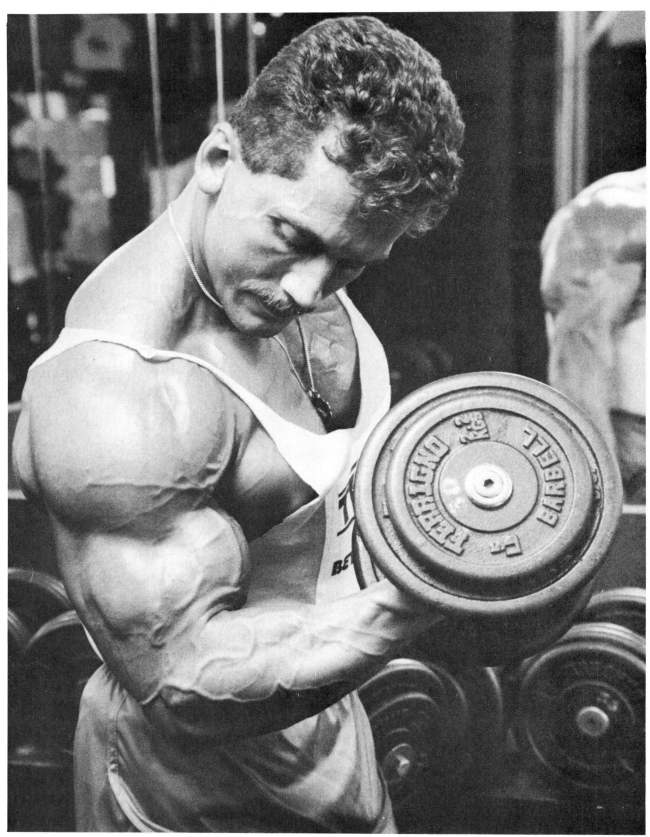

Night of Champions victor Lee Labrada does a set of alternate curls.

MIND OVER MATTER— POWER THINKING

Few people put real thinking power into their bodybuilding. Those who do go further and in a shorter period of time. It is true that more and more is being discovered about the mind. We know for sure that it's far more complicated than any computer man has invented. The beauty of the human mind is that we can learn to control it and make it work for us. This is especially true when it comes to bodybuilding. For example, a simple mental commitment to train can be made in a few seconds without saying a word. You merely tell yourself that you will train regularly for a certain time period, say six months or a year.

Goal setting is another mind game that you can put into your brain. Just as you can program a computer, you can program your mind to strive to reach certain goals.

Visualization and inspiration, too, are both controlled by the mind. With simple practice you can learn to "see" yourself as you want to be, and you can draw up inspiration by the bucketful.

Finally, there is concentration, the art of shutting everything out except the exercise you are doing at the time. Use this technique and you'll get more from your reps than ever before.

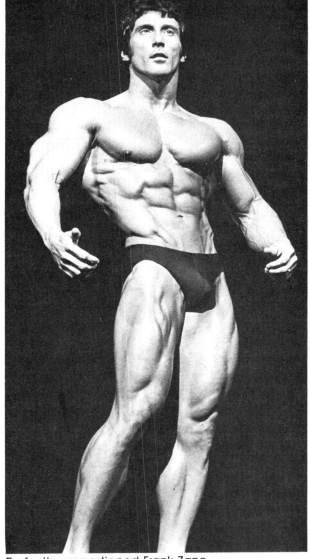

Perfectly proportioned Frank Zane.

41

CONCENTRATION

When you enter a hard-core training establishment like World Gym, one of the first things you become aware of is the enormous concentration people use when they are exercising. There's nothing fake about it, either. Successful bodybuilders know that the better their concentration, the more effort and feel they can promote, and, as a consequence, the more the muscle will be stressed.

Concentration begins with a mental picture of your individual muscles as they are being exercised. Stare down at your biceps when you are performing concentration curls. Watch the muscle react under the tension. *Will* the weight to rise up, and really *feel* the negative part of the movement as you lower the dumbbell to the arm-straight position. At first, full concentration may be difficult, but practice makes perfect.

When you perform multijoint movements, such as dips, presses, squats, etc., make a point of identifying the muscle you are trying to build. For example, the seated behind-neck press is a shoulder exercise, but it also works the back and triceps. For best results, however, you should concentrate on your shoulders while you perform the movement. The simple act of focusing on the deltoids and concentrating on involving them as much as possible in the lifting is a secret to bodybuilding success. Pinpoint your concentration the World Gym way and join the elite of bodybuilding.

GOAL SETTING

Haphazard training won't cut it! You need to set goals—achievable, realistic goals— to get ahead in this game. Having something to aim for gives your workouts purpose and meaning; both are essential ingredients if you want to better yourself in any field of endeavor.

You can set your long-term goals (most bodybuilders dream of becoming either Mr. or Ms. Olympia), but within your long-

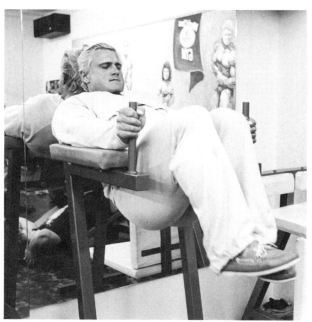

Tom Platz uses super concentration techniques to make every rep count.

term dream you should subdivide your desires into short-term, achievable goals that can be reached at 60–90 day intervals. After you reach each short-term goal, set your sights higher for something else. The Olympia? Yes, every dyed-in-the-wool bodybuilder's dream, yet it may not be within your grasp. Hope, pray, and train for it, but don't bank on it. Remember that Mr. Olympia or Ms. Olympia can be only one person each year, and, to complicate matters, bodybuilders such as Arnold Schwarzenegger, Lee Haney, and Cory Everson are so dominant in their development (much of it through genetic superiority—though I hasten to add by no means all) that they win the Olympia title over and over, which excludes new or upcoming bodybuilders from winning this top pro prize. Is an Olympia title in the cards for you? Well, you're fighting the odds, but someone has to win it, right?

Goal-setting athletes develop a healthy tunnel vision aimed at ultimate victory. This enables them to deal with training problems effectively as they arise. Under-par body parts are literally *attacked* every workout. Poor posing presentation turns into an *obsession* to find and coordinate the right music with the most skillful posing possible. Inferiority complexes are made use of to give us the determination to forge ahead. The superachievers in bodybuilding have programmed their bodies for success. They have set their minds on a particular target. They are totally confident in their ability to achieve it, and they persist relentlessly in their struggle.

What do you tell yourself before you begin a set? Invariably you decide how many reps you will do. You promise yourself a certain amount of willed intensity. You program your computer: "I'll do twelve reps," or "I'll go for seven superstrict reps and then do three cheating reps." The point is that if you don't set a demanding goal in a set, you won't push yourself to progress.

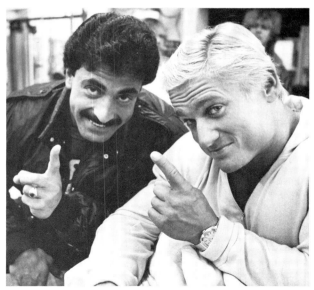

Samir and Tom both feel they're number one.

VISUALIZATION

I earnestly believe that correct visualization carries with it a power pack of magic. Right from the beginning Arnold Schwarzenegger visualized his biceps growing like bulging mountains. He visualized himself looking like Reg Park, his earliest and possibly his only hero. I have never known a man before or since Arnold who could *see* himself a bodybuilding success before it happened. And with seven Mr. Olympias under his belt, he called it a day and visualized himself as a box-office hit in the movies. There was never the slightest doubt in his mind that he would succeed. It's the same with his business ventures. Everything he touches turns to gold.

There is indisputable evidence to show that the way you visualize your performance before you actually attempt it greatly influences the result. For example, if you only half-believe you can make a lift, your chance of success is about 50 percent. If you have doubts about making the lift at all, then there is zero chance that you'll do it (not 10 percent or 5 percent chance . . . zero chance!). On the other hand, if you are *totally convinced* that you can lift that weight, there is zero chance you'll fail. That is the reality of the power of your mind.

Positive and vivid visualization excites the mind, turns on the adrenaline, clears the neural pathways, concentrates the effort, shuts out the interruption, taps the endorphins, puts your body in gear for an all-out effort, and guarantees success!

YOUR FIRST ROUTINE

I have given members of my gyms thousands of routines—beginner routines, intermediate routines, and advanced routines. Today I have instructors like Ed Giuliani and Zabo Kozewski to take over that job—unless you happen to be an extremely pretty woman. If that's the case, I just may be persuaded to help you out with your training now and again. Time permitting, of course.

Your body has seven different areas that need attention. I recommend that beginners perform just one exercise for each area. Exercises may be added as the weeks go by, but it is important that the beginner be introduced to weight training gently—with tender loving care. An early experience with too much weight or too many sets can turn you off for a lifetime. A total beginner who has never followed any formal exercise regime should at first perform only one set of each exercise. You can add more sets as the weeks go by. After a month, you can try three sets.

Here is the World Gym Beginner's Routine:

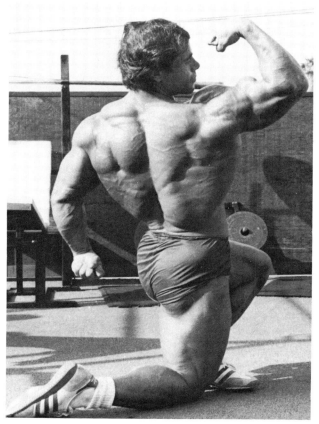

Franco flexes on the outdoor deck at World Gym.

Squats (legs)—20 repetitions. No weight.

Select a block of wood one to two inches thick; place only your heels on this block to maintain correct balance. Squat down until the upper side of your thigh is parallel to the floor. Return to the standing position and repeat. In due course you will perform this exercise with a barbell held across the back of your shoulders, after taking it from special support stands (squat racks).

During the movement it is necessary to keep your back flat, your seat stuck outward, and your head up. All squats should be performed either in front of a mirror or

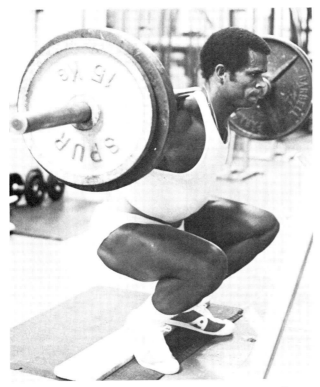

a plain wall. This avoids distraction from the buzzing activity of most gyms. Always wear a belt when performing squats with a barbell. Breathe in as you lower yourself into the deep knee bend position, and breathe out as you straighten your legs.

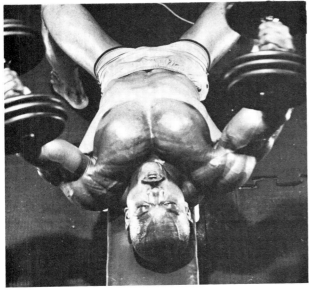

Dumbbell Bench Press (chest)— 12 repetitions.

Lie on your back on a flat bench with a loaded dumbbell in each hand. Keeping

your elbows out to the sides, press both dumbbells upward through a vertical path until your arms are straight. Lower and repeat. Do not bounce the weights on your chest. Press and lower at a moderate pace, always making sure you can lower the weights under control. Breathe in before you push up. Breathe out as your arms straighten. You may find it a little difficult at first to keep the dumbbells steady, but after two or three workouts you'll get this under control.

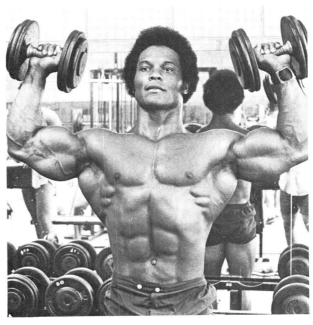

Dumbbell Press (shoulders)— 12 repetitions.

Stand with feet comfortably apart, holding a dumbbell in each hand at shoulder height. Hold your head up and lock your knees. Press the weights simultaneously above your head to the arms-straight position. Hold your elbows out to the sides as you do so. Lower and repeat. Do not lean backward as you press the weights up. Inhale before starting the lift. Exhale as your arms straighten.

Bent-Over Rows (back)— 12 repetitions.

Bend over at the waist, keeping your back flat and your knees slightly bent. Hold a dumbbell in each hand, hanging down at

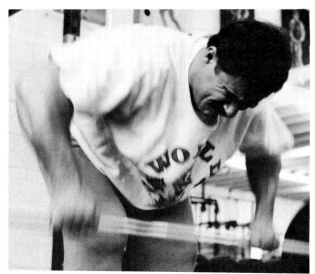

Bent-over rows build back width.

arm's length. Raise the dumbbells from the floor, pulling strongly into your waist area. Lower slowly, all the way down, stretching your lat muscles, and repeat. Keep your head up and your back flat throughout the exercise. Inhale before lifting. Exhale as the dumbbells reach your midsection.

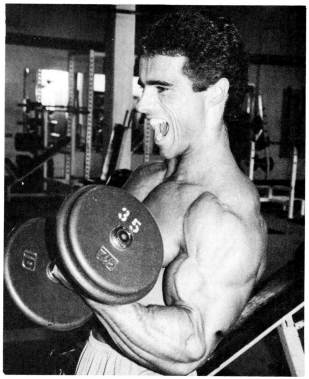

Newcomer Steve Brisbois executes a set of alternate dumbbell curls.

Dumbbell Curls (biceps)— 10 repetitions.

Stand with a pair of dumbbells in your hands, feet comfortably apart, arms down by your sides. Commence to curl the bells upward while keeping your upper arms tight against your torso. Lower and repeat under control. Do not "drop" the weights. Inhale before curling. Exhale as the dumbbells reach their highest point.

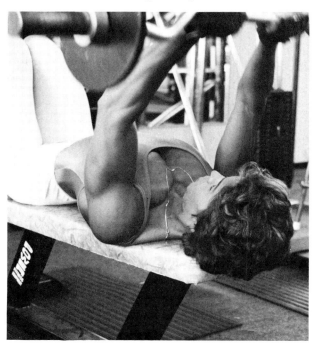

Triceps Extensions (triceps)— 12 repetitions.

Lie on your back on a flat exercise bench. Hold a light barbell at arm's length overhead. Lower the weight slowly by bending the elbows, striving to keep the upper arms vertical throughout the exercise. Lower the bar to the top of your nose, being extremely careful not to actually hit your nose in the process. Raise and repeat. Inhale before lowering. Exhale as the arms straighten.

Roman Chair Sit-Ups (abdominals)— 20 repetitions.

Sit on a Roman chair apparatus, making sure that your feet are properly secured. Place your hands on your lap or on your

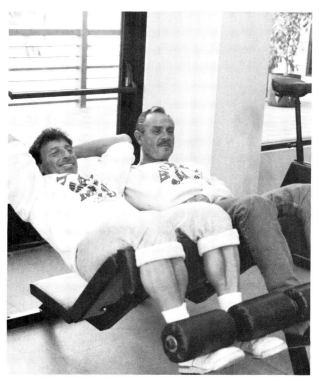

Eddie and Zabo training their abs.

waist. Recline slowly until your torso is parallel to the floor. Rise and repeat. Breathe in before starting to recline. Breathe out as you complete the sit-up.

WHAT POUNDAGE?

No one can tell you what poundage you should use in your exercises. The important thing is that you perform the exercises as directed—without strain. Always train well within your means. Later, as you really get into your workouts, you will be able to increase the poundage so that your muscles are challenged on a regular basis. As a beginner you should never give

in to the temptation to cheat in your exercises. No bouncing, tossing, or swinging.

WARMING UP

Warm-ups are important. It's a good idea to run on the spot, ride a stationary bike, or jump rope for a few minutes before training. This will get the heart pumping and get you ready, willing, and able to do your weight training.

Whether you are a beginning, intermediate, or advanced trainer, your first set of each exercise should be done with less than maximum weight. For example, a person able to perform three sets of 10 repetitions with 100 pounds in the curl exercise should warm up with one set of about 15 repetitions with about 60 pounds.

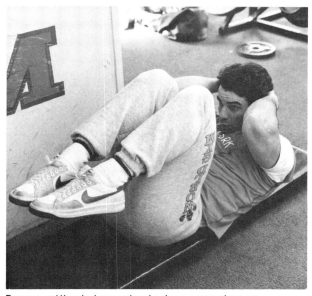

Proper attire is important when warming up.

SHAPE TRAINING— BALANCING AND BUILDING

Hitting the sets and reps is important. You've got to get a lot under your belt to come out a winner. I'm no advocate of the so-called heavy-duty method of training. To me all bodybuilding is heavy duty. Intensity *is* an important factor, but it is most definitely not the only factor in gaining muscle mass. Two sets per exercise is not enough, however much effort is used. People who know me often have definite opinions about what makes me tick. None of those opinions, however, even hint that I do not speak my mind; nor that I do not speak the truth as I see it. I'll say it again: *Two sets of an exercise, however intense, will not build an Olympian-winning physique!* It's not my way—nor any champion's way that I have observed.

If you are inclined to try heavy duty, or any other form of training, then do so. You will doubtless learn something. Experimentation is good, so don't get the idea that I'm trying to dissuade you from finding things out for yourself.

My training philosophy is to work each muscle group from a variety of angles; to use any style it takes to get the muscle stressed; to increase intensity levels periodically, and then back cycle to hold onto gains. Quality training must go hand in hand with a positive mental attitude. Your workout pace must be businesslike, neither too slow nor too rushed. And each workout must be linked to proper goal-setting phases.

World Gym is *not* a powerlifting establishment, although we have scores of extremely strong men and women. World's is for muscle building. That is our business. It was my original concept, and it will be my last. I am interested in building and shaping the body.

In fact, the main difference between a champion and an also-ran is shape. For every superstar champion that trains at

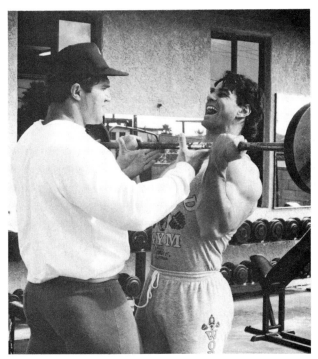

Gary Strydom helps Jon-Jon Park with a set of barbell curls.

World Gym, there are a dozen more who are bigger (and stronger). But they lack that magic ingredient: shape.

Genetics goes a long way toward forming your shape. Not too many people will deny the extraordinary natural shape of trainers like Cory Everson, Rachel McLish, Jon-Jon Park, Danny Padilla, Lee Haney, Gary Strydom, or Bob Paris. But there are others with a little less natural shape who have become just as shapely and awesomely impressive. The purpose of shape training is to develop a balanced and symmetrical physique. In this day, more than ever before, it is vitally important. I have made capsulized comments about changing shape for the better in the various body parts. Don't neglect shape training. It's the thing that title winners do that also-rans fail to do.

SHOULDERS

If you're round-shouldered, or appear to be flat at the back of your shoulders, you must put in plenty of work for the posterior deltoids. Bent-over laterals done with dumbbells or pulleys are among the best exercises for this area. You will notice that those bodybuilders who do lots of bent-over rowing movements, ostensibly for the lats, invariably have good posterior deltoids. There are also specific machines that are designed just for the rear delt area. Cybex makes an excellent model.

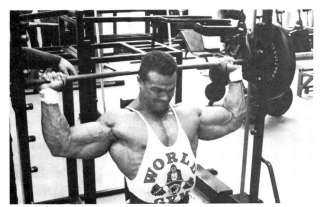

Perfect form with behind-the-neck presses can help you achieve Olympian shoulder development as demonstrated here by Brad Verret.

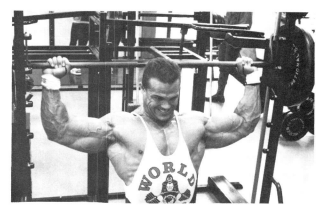

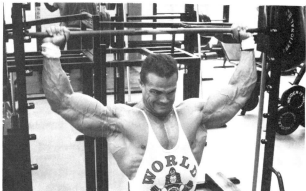

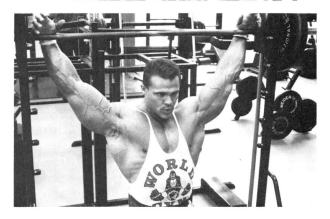

The side deltoids contribute to impressive shoulder width. You just cannot be too big here. Concentrate on dumbbell and pulley lateral raises. The behind-neck press, especially in the seated position with the elbows held back as much as possible, also works the side delts. Don't forget to experiment with your repetition counts in this excellent exercise. My experience has shown that good results can come from heavy weights, if you use just five reps, or lower weights if you go all the way up to twenty reps per set. Mix up your reps and keep your shoulders guessing.

The frontal shoulder area is usually pretty well built from bench-pressing with barbells and dumbbells, but you still need to perform some isolation work to keep the front delts separated from the pectorals. Unlike in the "old days," judges do not look for "tie-in" anymore. They look for muscle separation, where one muscle group is defined distinctively from another.

BICEPS

Shaping the biceps is difficult. It can be done, but you will not totally transform them. In other words, if you have a flat, *peakless* arm, no amount of effort will give you Schwarzenegger-peaked biceps.

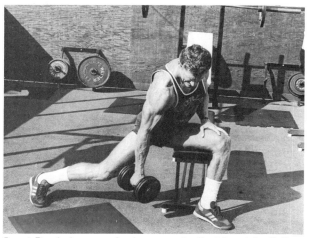

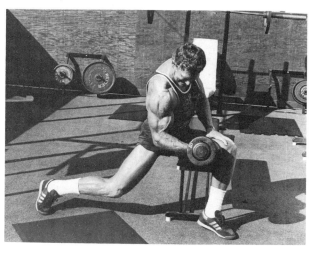

Brad Davis is a perfect example that bodybuilding can help maintain a young, energetic, healthy look. Here he demonstrates one of his favorite exercises, the concentration curl.

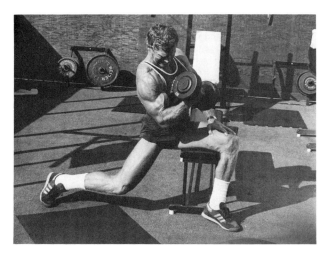

Concentration curls will help, as will regular posing and cramping. You should also make a point of strongly flexing your biceps at the top of every curl. Yes, every rep.

For those of you who have an overabundance of *gap* between your biceps and your forearm when you flex up, I suggest plenty of reverse curls (holding the barbell with the palms down) and hammer curls (curling dumbbells with the palms facing each other, thumbs uppermost).

You should also perform plenty of preacher-bench curls with the bench platform set at a shallow angle (30–35 degrees). Use barbells or dumbbells for this movement.

THE BACK

The back can be divided into several different areas—the trapezius, the lower back, the upper back, and the middle back. The challenge is to build both back width and back thickness.

The Trapezius

Want traps like those of Mike Christian or Serge Nubret? Perform plenty of dumbbell or barbell shrugs. You can also do these on the Universal machine, which has a weight stack for convenient changing of weight load.

Building Back Width

You can't build too much back spread. It gives you that all-important "V" shape.

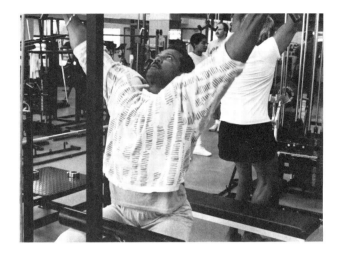
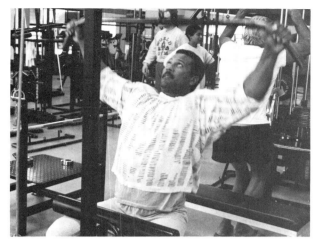
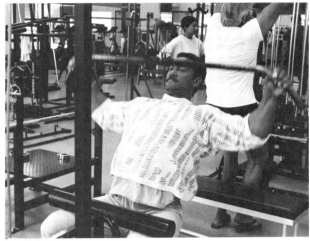
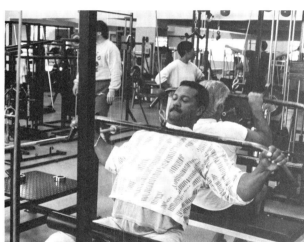

Wide grip lat pulldowns are a fundamental exercise toward building a wide, wing-like back. Here is a perfect rep of the exercise demonstrated by Manny Perry.

Don't neglect wide-grip chins; almost every champion I know uses them. Lat pulldowns, using a wide grip, are also a wideback builder. The scapulae are actually stretched and pulled outward, leading to that much desired "V" appearance.

Building a Thicker Back

Few exercises build a thick back quicker than bent-over rowing, but there's a lot to be said for the regular use of power cleans and even deadlifts. If you find that rowing with a barbell is too hard on your lower back, switch to T-bar rows or even rows on a special apparatus in which the torso is supported in the prone (face-down) position.

Lower Back

Deadlifts build this section in a superior way. Don't push the poundages too high. And never bounce the barbell on the floor or from a platform. Back sufferers should consider prone hyper-extensions as a substitute for deadlifts and other potentially aggravating lower-back movements.

Middle Back

Sit on the floor and, using a low pulley, draw the pulley handles into your waistline area. At the moment when you cannot pull back any farther, press your shoulder blades together vigorously and squeeze the central area of the back with as much intensity as possible. Do this with each repetition.

THIGHS

Like the back, the thighs have several distinctly different sections that may require special training techniques to bring about good shape and a balanced appearance.

Upper Thighs

This area seldom needs special attention. The upper thigh is usually the first part to grow when leg exercises are done. The regular back squat with a barbell across your shoulders will give you all the upper-thigh development you'll need.

Lower Thighs

This part of the thigh can often prove difficult to build, especially for people with long legs. Back squats do not always build lower thighs. Concentrate more on exercises such as hack lifts, sissy squats, and Smith machine squats (with feet forward of body).

Outer Thigh Sweep

Regular back squats usually contribute greatly to giving a good outer sweep, but if you are having a problem, try hack slides with feet and knees close together. Leg presses can be performed in the same way.

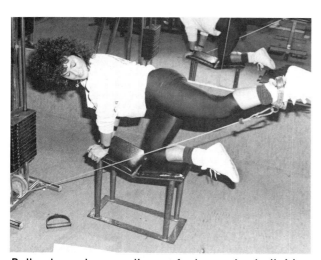

Pulley leg raises are the perfect exercise to tighten the glutes.

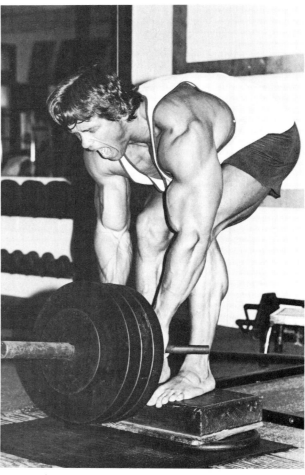

Arnold Schwarzenegger performs T-bar rows.

Inner Thighs

Perform hack slides and squats with your feet facing outward and with your legs spread wide, out to the sides. Inner thighs can also be worked effectively with special inner-leg machines, or by using pulleys whereby the legs are drawn together against resistance.

Thigh Biceps

There's little doubt that some bodybuilders just don't have a natural thigh biceps. They have to sweat blood to build the area. Try both standing and lying thigh curls. Some people find they get a better *feel* by using a dumbbell held between the feet. If all else fails, try a large number of sets (10) with high reps (15–20).

ABDOMINALS

Building abdominals that show is not just a matter of a good waist-trimming exercise program. You need to reduce overall calories, especially foods high in fat, to thin your skin enough to get the layers of abdominals to show up clearly.

Problem upper abdominals can be built with crunches and Roman chair sit-ups. Lower abs, however, are usually the tricky area to build up. The best exercises for this part of the midsection include hanging leg raises (legs straight or bent) or knee tucks while lying or sitting on an exercise bench.

TRICEPS

The best building exercises for the triceps are the close grip bench press, the parallel bar dip, and the lying triceps stretch. The problem with the triceps is that usually it doesn't develop enough in the lower part. To correct this you should perform plenty of bent-over dumbbell kickbacks. Be aware, however, that if you have a "high" triceps, with few muscle cells in the lower area, you will not be able to change the condition with any exercise or combination or exercises.

CALVES

Lower legs are frequently a problem. Combine donkey calf raises with heavy standing calf raises. In the latter exercise use both low reps (8–10) and high reps (20–25).

If you have poor inner-calf development, perform your calf raises with the toes

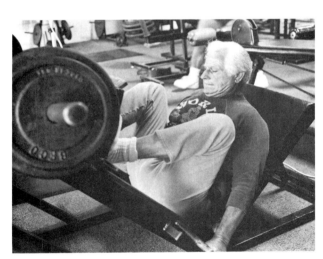

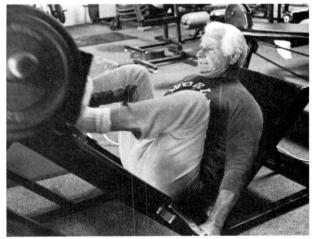

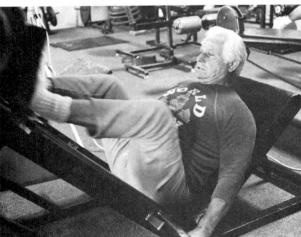

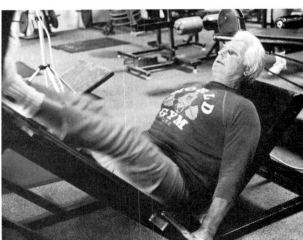

Joe Gold performs a perfect set of 45-degree leg presses.

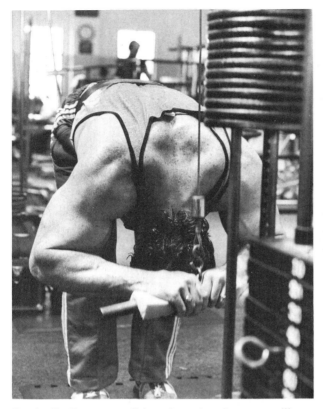

Rocky DeFerro uses this unique bent-over position to perform his tricep extensions. By looking at his arms who could argue with this technique?

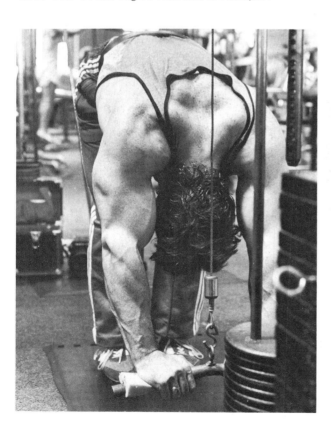

pointed outward. Those with poor outer-calf development should perform their calf raises with the toes pointed inward. If you have no problem with inner/outer balance, perform your calf raises with the feet facing straight forward, keeping the main stress over the big toe.

FOREARMS

Reverse curls and hammer curls are great forearm builders. Use high-rep wrist curls to build the belly of your forearms. Forearms can be worked advantageously three times a week instead of the standard two times. The best advice I can offer for those who have under-par forearms is to work them at the beginning of the workout. Because almost every weight-training exercise we do involves the forearms, by working them first we preexhaust them. As a result, they will be stressed heavily during the balance of the workout. Expect more growth!

THE CHEST

You can build up different parts of your chest. For maximum impressiveness the best areas to focus on are the upper and outer sections of the pectorals. Generally speaking, you should study your own chest development and train the weaker areas with more sets and intensity.

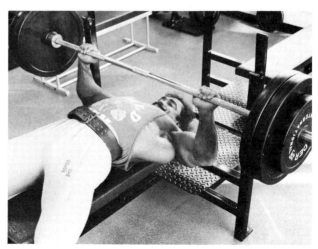

A staple exercise for chest development—the bench press.

Upper Pecs

All incline presses and flyes work the upper part of the chest. The best incline angle is 30–40 degrees. Anything steeper than that will work the front delts to the exclusion of the pectorals.

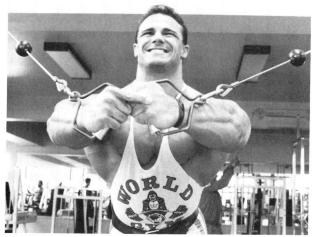

Cable crunches for a well-developed chest.

Lower Pecs

Decline flyes and decline barbell and dumbbell presses will bring the lower pecs into play. Beware, however, of building too much lower pec. You need enough lower pec to define the bottom pec line (even when the arm is raised in a double biceps pose), but that's it. Do not build more than is needed.

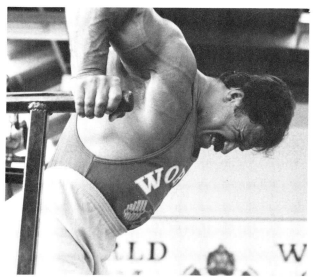

Ali Malla performs parallel dips for lower chest development.

Outer Pecs

Add width to your pecs and you will look doubly impressive! It will make your waist look smaller and your torso look wider. The best exercise for the outer pecs is wide-grip parallel bar dips, elbows out, chin on chest, feet forward. Supine flyes also contribute extensively to outer pectoral development.

Inner Pecs

Close-grip bench presses done in flat and incline positions will help. Probably the best two exercises for the inner pecs are Pek-Dek flyes and cable crossovers. You should conclude each rep with a conscious flex of the inner pec area, just to let your chest know which area you want to build.

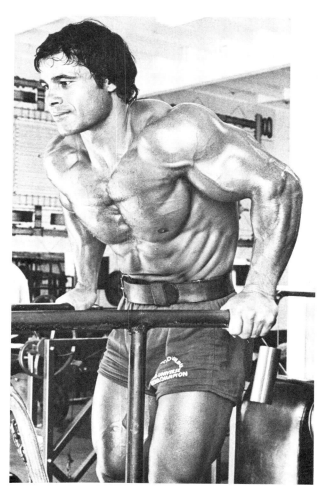

Franco in peak condition.

HARD-CORE TRAINING STRATEGIES—PRINCIPLES OF PROGRESS

Planned training always works best. I'm convinced of it. You'll find that some principles don't work for you while others bring remarkable results, but even so it's always good to have a plan, a special method to follow. There is always a degree of trial and error in bodybuilding, and it never ends. You are forever experimenting; that's the nature of bodybuilding.

Progress in bodybuilding comes *fastest* for beginners, who have never lifted weights before, and for seasoned bodybuilders who have enjoyed a prolonged layoff from training. The reason, of course, is that workouts suddenly surprise the body with their intensity, most noticeably for those who haven't trained before, or at least who haven't trained in a long while. But there's more to the story! After increasing like crazy for a while, your growth rate will slow down and may finally stop altogether. You can add sets, push harder in your reps, eat more, rest better—but the answer is always: sticking point. Nothing happens. Your muscles just do not want to grow bigger. Don't be unduly concerned. Sticking points are natural; 95 percent of all bodybuilders have them.

Bodybuilding with weights and machines is stressful, and when you subject your body to this form of physical stress it

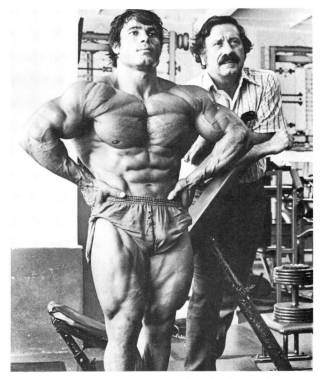

Franco Columbu and Joe Weider in the early years.

reacts by preparing for more of the same. Muscles and tendons strengthen and enlarge. In subsequent workouts this overcompensation continues, but there comes a time when your body will no longer continue to add muscle and size unless there is a *very* good reason. Merely repeating what you did to stress your body originally is often not enough to keep your muscles growing. New stresses and shocks have to be found.

Actually, sticking points are OK. There

have to be periods of slow or nonexistent growth so that the muscles can consolidate their gains; sometimes a little size may even be lost. Nevertheless, look upon sticking points with some degree of tolerance. They are plateaus at which your body is taking stock, building a base from which to leap to the *next* level of muscular achievement. Your job is to see that sticking points are neither too frequent nor last too long.

Conceding that muscles are jolted into growth with new high-intensity stimulus, it might seem elementary that all we have to do is "shock" the muscles each workout to keep them growing. Theoretically this is true, but it does not work out in reality. Let's say a person with stubborn calf development performs five sets of 25 reps twice a week; it's obvious those same calves could be "shocked" if he were suddenly to hit them with a hundred sets. But would growth result? No. The result would be bed for a week! The art then is to shock the muscles into growth, but not so much as to overtrain them and not allow them to recuperate in a reasonable time.

To shock their muscles into growth bodybuilders have tried everything in the book. All-day training of one body part has been tried. Not recommended. Performing an entirely different routine each workout has been attempted. Not recommended. Working the *same* body part with high intensity every day, ten days in a row, has been done. Not recommended. Eating a half chicken every hour, on the hour . . . not recommended. The madness goes on—and strength and muscle mass are *not* among the benefits.

Arnold Schwarzenegger had the workable middle-of-the-road approach: "I change around my exercises from time to time, and even perform them in a different manner—to shock my muscles into growing."

Performing the same exercises, sets, and reps leads to boredom. Variety, properly balanced, will bring about reaction.

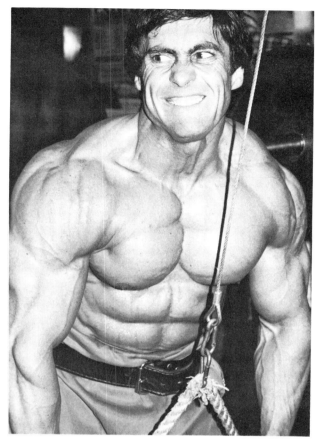

French star Jacques Neuville does tricep pressdowns and in so doing shows incredible cuts and ab development.

Your job is to ascertain just *when* your muscles need to be shocked, and to what degree. Obviously, if you are adding poundage (while maintaining good form), you are making progress. No need at this time to get into shocking the muscles. Wait until you hit the sticking point before you get into the tricky stuff. It is when the fullest intensity has been applied to a muscle that you need to get out your shock-training notebook. You must, in some devious manner, overwhelm your stubborn muscles with a complete change of pace, a new exercise, considerably more or fewer repetitions, a change in exercise style or sequence, or in the frequency of your workouts. But all the time you have to walk that fine line between stimulation for growth and overstimulation for entrenchment into the dreaded sticking point.

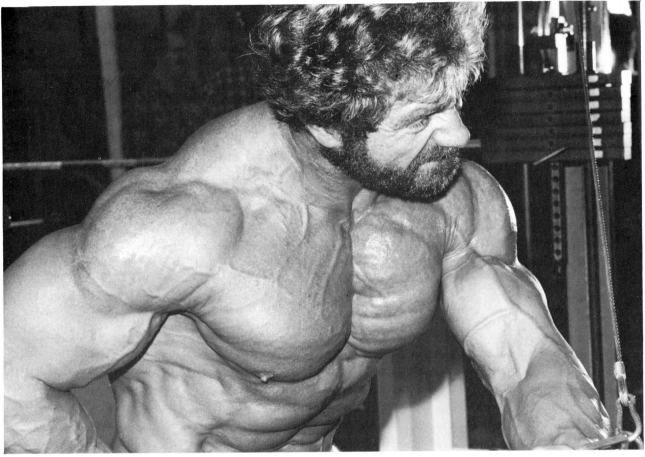

Jusup Wilcosz.

DIMINISHING SETS

Apply this principle to any series of exercises. The methodology of diminishing sets is to race the clock while keeping intensity in your workout. This double incentive serves to increase muscle size like you wouldn't believe. The idea is to perform 100 reps of an exercise in as few sets as possible, with rest time between sets at a minimum. First time out, you will probably need to do several sets to do 100 reps—as many as 10. Gradually cut down to four sets, at which time you should increase your poundage.

Don't worry about performing four even sets of 25 reps each. The first set may be 40 reps, 30 for the second, 20 for the third, and 10 for the fourth and last. Squeeze out as many reps as you can in every set. Don't baby yourself in those early sets for a better performance later on.

Diminishing sets will give a new pump to your muscles—and in order to meet the challenge they will grow.

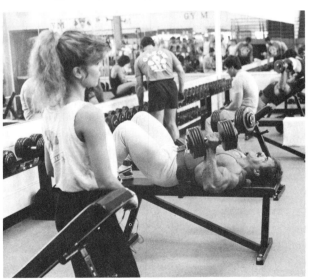

Another good chest builder are flat-bench flyes as perform by Ali Malla.

COMPOUND SETS

This method is also known in Weiderese as Giant Sets. It is definitely an advanced way of training and should not be used by beginners or those who have only been in the sport a few months.

A compound set is the consecutive performance of four or five exercises for one body part, followed by a brief rest period.

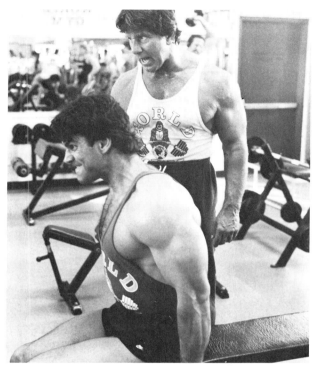

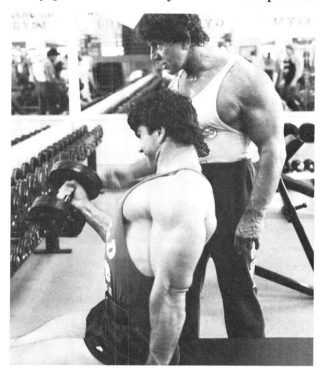

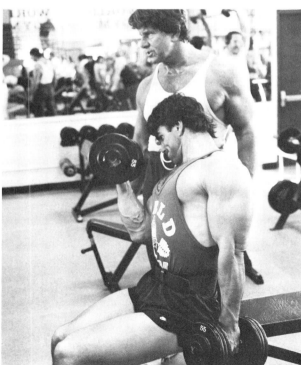

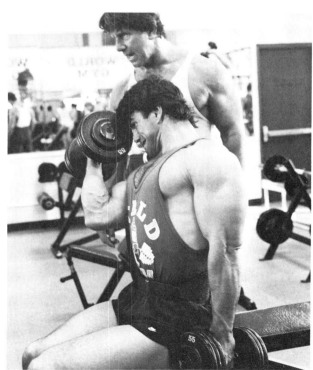

Seated alternate curls performed by Jon-Jon Park as his father Reg stands over him making sure he gets everything out of his set.

For instance, an entire thigh routine might be the following (which should be performed three times):

Compound Set	Reps
Regular Squat	10
Hack Lift	12
Leg Press	10
Thigh Extension	12
Rest (three minutes)	

The following is a compound set for the triceps (performed three times):

Compound Set	Reps
Close-Grip Bench Press	8
Lying Triceps Extension	10
Parallel Bar Dips	10
Standing Triceps Extensions	12
Triceps Pressdowns	15
Rest (two minutes)	

Bob Paris, who trains at the World Gym, often used this method of training and obtained excellent results. When he trained his legs in this way few people could follow him through a workout, because he went from one exercise to another with absolutely no rest.

SUPERSETS

A superset is the alternation of two exercises for opposing muscle groups with a minimum amount of rest. Typical supersets involve alternating a triceps and a biceps movement, or alternating Roman chair sit-ups with prone hyperextensions. Actually, the term superset is used so loosely today it can refer to the alternation of *any* two exercises, whether they are from opposing muscle groups or not. Accordingly, alternating two types of curls could be called a superset, although in the purest definition of the word this would not qualify as such.

Supersets may not build more strength than straight sets, but they do help a bodybuilder train faster, get a better pump, and increase stress factors on the muscles being blitzed. This can lead to additional growth over a relatively short

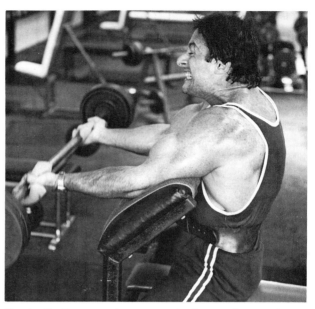

Rocky DeFerro works on a set of preacher curls.

period of time. Supersets, especially if two-handed exercises are practiced, can also save a bodybuilder valuable time, because they bring about quicker muscle fatigue than other methods. They can also improve fitness levels because of increased cardiovascular efficiency, as well as aiding in the fat-burning process.

DESCENDING SETS

In Britain they call this method the triple drop. Arnold Schwarzenegger frequently used this technique when training his biceps. He calls it the "stripping" method. A descending set, as the name implies, involves the reduction of weight during the performance of an exercise. This is done when you can no longer continue a set.

Take the barbell curl as an example. You start curling with, say, 120 pounds. You manage five or six difficult reps. When you can't do any more, two partners slide off a disk from either end. Now, with a barbell 20 to 30 pounds lighter, you can continue for several more repetitions. Again, when you can do no more, two more disks are removed, and you keep pumping until you reach normal failure.

It is vital that disks be removed simultaneously, with care, yet with utmost speed. Don't rest after your training partners have taken off the weights.

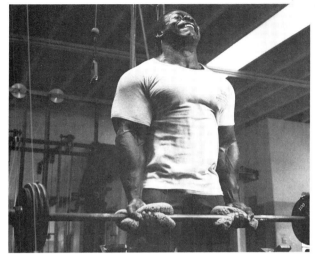

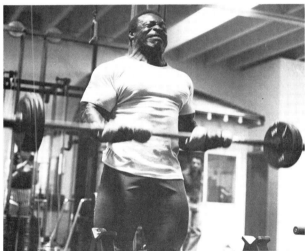

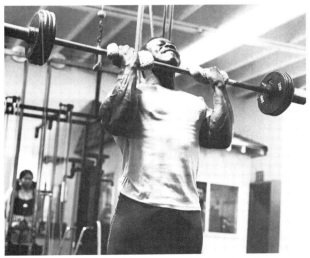

Roy Callender has his own perfect style of performing the barbell curl.

Most exercises lend themselves to this technique. If you are using a machine that has a selection pin, reducing the resistance is that much simpler. Only one training partner is required to pull out the pin and insert it at a lesser weight. With some machines you can do it yourself.

This stripping method is one of the most severe of all. Dynamic Tom Platz uses it frequently. Perform fewer overall sets than you would normally, otherwise you could overtrain and fail to recuperate in time for your next workout.

TRISETS

As the name suggests, you will be using three different exercises in the triset technique. Perform one after the other with no rest in between. You may rest for a couple of minutes after the triset—then repeat the whole process. Trisets are usually performed three or four times and can be used in two distinct ways. You may use the multiangular approach, in which different sections of a muscle are worked so that maximum size is achieved in all areas, or you may use the uniangular method to blitz just one section—the lower thighs, for instance.

As an example of hitting a muscle from three different angles, let's take the deltoids (shoulders). First perform the bentover flyes for the rear deltoid; then the side deltoid can be hit with the standard lateral-raise exercise; and finally the front delts can be stimulated with alternate front raises with dumbbells. In a similar manner, different sections of the biceps can be hit with preacher curls, barbell curls, and concentration curls.

The uniangular triset is even more lethal. You are stressing the same part of a muscle with three exercises.

Take the lower thighs, often a problem area. A suitable triset could consist of sissy squats, hack slides, and thigh extensions. Few other methods would stimulate the lower thighs into growth as well as this technique.

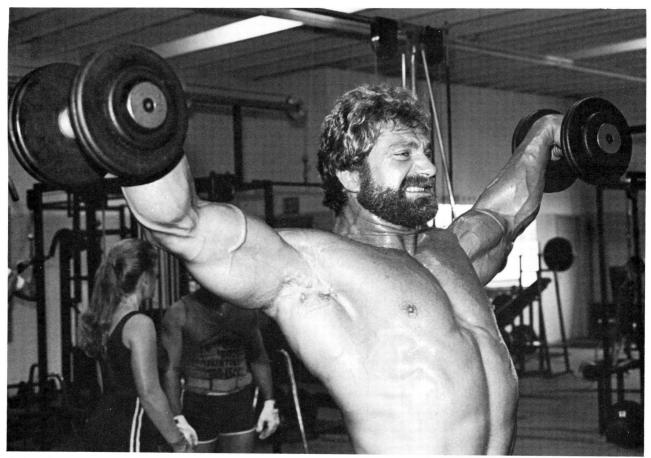

Jusup Wilcosz performs a perfect rep of lateral raises.

THE PREEXHAUST METHOD

This method is relatively new, but certainly it is used today by a host of bodybuilders all over the world. Like most blitz or specialized techiques the preexhaust method was not designed for extensive off-season use. It is a quickie solution to problem areas that refuse to grow. I do not feel it should be used longer than about five to eight weeks, not because of any danger to health or chance of injury, but because too much of a good thing (excessive stimulation) can lead to burnout.

Preexhaust is the battering of a specific muscle with a carefully chosen *isolation* exercise, followed immediately by a *combination* movement. Let's use the shoulders as an example. As you may know, the triceps is the "weak link" involved in many shoulder exercises. In essence, when you perform standing presses with dumb-

bells or barbells the triceps is worked hard and the deltoids themselves may be worked only moderately. The more effort you put into your shoulder presses, the quicker the triceps tires, yet you're still not really fatiguing the deltoids. You have to get around the weak link triceps, and the only way to do this is to first preexhaust the shoulders with *isolation* exercises, such as dumbbell or pulley lateral raises; the triceps is not involved in this action and remains fresh and strong.

After a hard set of lateral raises that get you to the point of failure, proceed *immediately* to a combination movement, such as the behind-neck press. The triceps will now be considerably stronger than the preexhausted deltoids, so in essence those delts will be doubly pounded. The strong triceps demands the delt's fullest cooperation, which means more deltoid fiber is being worked. The following exercise combinations make useful preexhaust programs:

PREEXHAUST PROGRAMS

Isolation	Combination
Forearms	
Reverse wrist curl	Reverse curl
Calves	
Toe raise (leg-press machine)	Rope jumping
	High rebounder jump
Standing calf raise	
Donkey calf raise	
Rear Shoulders	
Bent-over flye	Bent-over barbell row
Bent-over cable flye	Seated cable row
Pek-Dek (reverse position)	
Side Shoulders	
Lateral raise	Upright row (wide grip)
Cable side raise	Behind-neck press
Back	
Nautilus pullover	Bent-over row
Barbell pullover	Chin to chest
Parallel bar shrugs	T-bar row
Trapezius	
Shrugs (barbell, dumbbell, calf machine, or bench)	Upright row
	Smith Machine clean
Thighs	
Leg extension	Squat
Roman chair squats	Front squat
	Hack slide
Chest	
Flat flye	Supine bench press
Pulley crossover	Dumbbell bench press
Pek-Dek flye	
Upper Chest	
Incline flye	Incline bench press
	Incline dumbbell press
Lower Chest	
Decline flye	Wide-grip parallel bar dip
Decline cable crossover	Decline bench press (barbell or dumbbell)
Thigh Biceps	
Lying leg curl (machine)	Upside-down squat (with gravity boots)
Standing leg curl	
Waist	
Crunch	Hanging leg raise
	Inverted sit-up (with gravity boots)

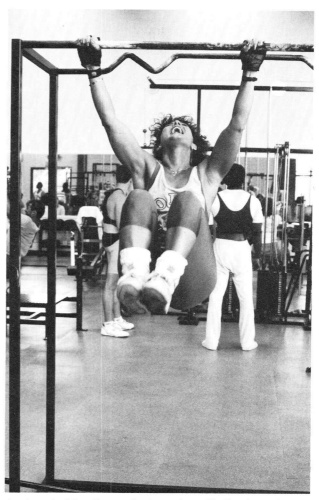

Andrea LaMantia works her abs with the hanging knee raise.

PYRAMID TRAINING

Experienced bodybuilders (that's another way of saying *older* bodybuilders) often gravitate toward pyramid training. This method is widely used because it permits you to start into your sets easily, build to a peak, and taper off effectively.

Start with an initial set of high reps (12–15) using a light weight. Add weight for the next set and perform about 10 reps. This is done with each set until only a few reps are possible. Now it's time to "come down" the other side of the pyramid. Decrease the weight load significantly and increase your reps again. One more time, more reps still—and dump off even more disks. Pyramid routines are almost always used by champion bodybuilders on heavy exercises like squats, bench presses, rows, deadlifts, and shoulder presses. A typical pyramid routine for the bench press might look like this:

PYRAMID BENCH PRESS

Set 1	20 reps	120 lbs.
Set 2	10 reps	150 lbs.
Set 3	8 reps	170 lbs.
Set 4	6 reps	190 lbs.
Set 5	6 reps	210 lbs.
Set 6	3 reps	230 lbs.
Set 7	8 reps	140 lbs.
Set 8	15 reps	120 lbs.

Not everybody wants to go all the way to a Mr. Olympia title. There are heck of a lot of you out there who just want to shape up and look fit and dynamic—rock hard! In short, you want a steelworker's body.

Well, I've got news for you, and don't doubt my words: *It matters not whether you want 16-inch muscular arms and a steelworker's body, or 21-inch, contest-winning guns and a Mr. Olympia title; you have to train in exactly the same way, with superhard, intense workouts and correct nutritional practices. By no means do you get off easier because you only want a beach body!*

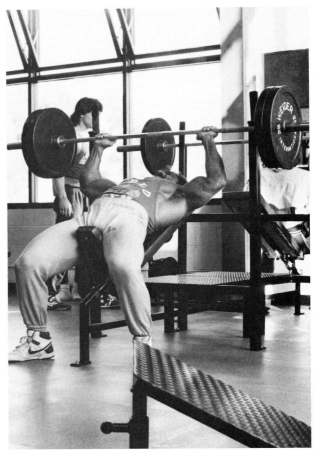

Incline barbell presses are great for upper chest development.

SOMETHING NEW—
EMPIRICAL TRAINING

I have watched more top bodybuilders train than any other person on Earth! Admittedly, that's a pretty wild claim—but it's true. There are plenty of similarities in the way champions train, but it seems to me that each one has picked up little idiosyncrasies, tricks if you like. A few bodybuilders, men like Serge Nubret, Al Beckles, and Tom Platz, train in totally unorthodox ways. But even so, sometimes I think there's not enough experimentation going on. Don't get me wrong—I'm in favor of bodybuilding basics, but as a champion climbs the ladder to Olympian success I feel it's to his or her advantage to try out new methods and techniques. Let's face it, you've got to do something to keep those muscles growing, and it is hitting them from different angles with variations of intensity that will do it. When you do experiment with different methods, make sure you take careful notes. You should never have to try the same experiment twice. If a new technique fails to give results after a six-week period, drop it like a hot potato.

One unusual and seldom-used method that is practiced by Sergio Oliva and Tom Platz is to perform a set of repetitions, and then at the point of rep failure, halt the set but don't put the weight on the rack or on the floor. At this point oxygen load by hyperventilating for more energy, but

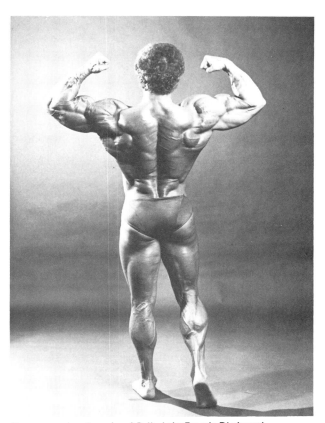

The massive back of Britain's Frank Richard.

while you do this, the burn is still there because the resistance is still around. Platz uses this method with all kinds of exercises, especially his biceps curls and his triceps pressdowns. It's not dissimilar to the rest-pause method, but in the case of rest-pause the resistance is usually racked for a few seconds.

Typically when Oliva does his seated calf raises he will stop two or three times

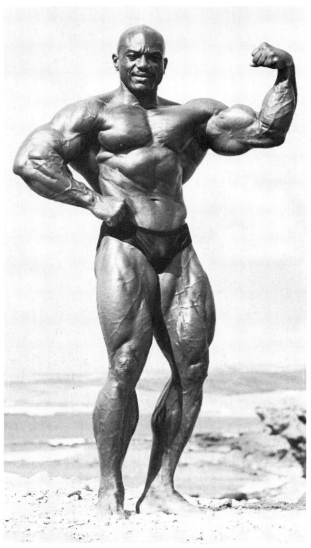

The unbelievable Sergio Oliva.

during the set, load oxygen, and then proceed to another failure (or near failure) point.

Serge Nubret, one of the most original trainers I've ever met, performs set after set of one-arm exercises, using high reps. He alternates arms, but attempts to perform one more rep each successive set. This *really* challenges both his intensity and endurance. But it works. To my knowledge, no other star bodybuilder has tried his training methods for any period of time. Serge especially enjoys this method when working his arms in the seated concentration-curl exercise and his shoulders in the lying lateral raise.

I'm not necessarily recommending that you try these methods. They just may not be compatible with your level of fitness or recuperative powers. What I am saying is that if you are at a sticking point in a particular body part, don't be afraid to try something unorthodox. Dare to be different!

I'm the last person to recommend that you overwork a muscle, but let's face facts: Arnold Schwarzenegger, whose biceps development has yet to be equalled, performed 30 sets just for that one muscle while in his teens. It was this admittedly crazy training that gave him the biggest and highest-peaked muscles in the world. This raises the question of whether or not muscle cells can be increased in number (hyperplasia). Scientists tell us we keep the number of muscle cells we were born with and that progressive resistance exercise merely enlarges each fiber. But there is some medical evidence to indicate that extremely hard training can cause muscle cells to split and multiply. Is this what Arnold did with this 30 sets of biceps exercise? It doesn't sound unreasonable to me.

How about those few bodybulders who stop a couple of times during a repetition for what are known as "contracted holds"? Obviously this wouldn't work well for all exercises, because some movements are almost impossible to control, but it can work pretty well for triceps pressdowns, lateral raises, curls, calf raises, flyes, crossover pulleys, Pek-Dek crunches, etc. It's not compatible with heavy power moves such as cleans, squats, bench presses, etc. What do "contracted holds" do for your development? Well, they introduce a new form of intensity to your workouts. Whether this will mean additional growth can only be determined by trying them yourself. I will say this, however: *It is those small increases in intensity, especially when made on a regular basis, that trigger muscle growth!*

Another method that I saw one of my gym members use on his lateral raises was to drop and catch the weights during

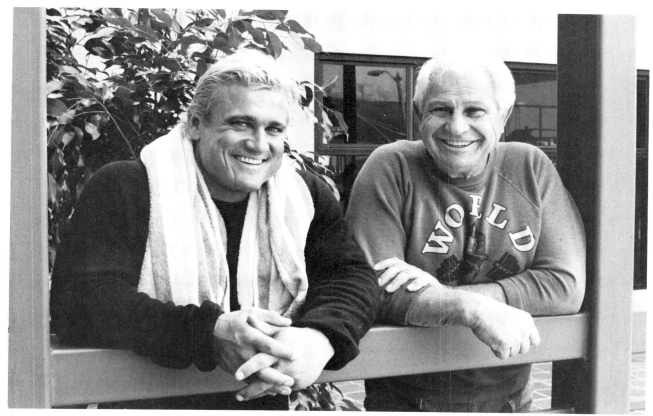

Tom Platz has been a good friend for years.

a set. Let me explain. He would use only moderate-to-light dumbbells. He would raise them in the normal lateral-raise fashion, but take them to a "10 past 10" clock position. From here he would drop his arms, releasing deltoid control of the dumbbells but "catching" and controlling the downward momentum when his arms reached the crucifix (arms parallel to the floor) position. He would repeat this for every rep of the set. It doesn't take a genius to figure out that one could be inviting trouble when playing with momentum. It is essential that you be an experienced trainer, and that you have practiced the movement regularly before trying this "catching" procedure. The last thing you want is a strained or torn muscle.

I often noticed that natural mesomorphs (those who are naturally muscular from day one) can gain from almost any type of regular routine, but endomorphs (fatties) and ectomorphs (skinnies) have to use specialized and planned routines to bring about regular gains. Making gains over and beyond the norm is usually achieved only with some form of increased intensity. This often involves a set taking longer than normal. When the average person stops a set and puts the weight on the floor, a superachieving bodybuilder will be just beginning.

Try the following to increase overall growth potential: when doing standing lateral raises, after reaching momentary failure, carry on the set by continuing with either dumbbell upright rows or standing presses, using the same weights as you did in the lateral raises and with no pause whatever when converting from laterals to presses. The same can be done with lying or incline flyes. As you come to a point where you can do no more, quickly change from the flye motion to the dumbbell press movement. It keeps the muscle screaming for help and growing from the added intensity-burn. Ouch!

A little imagination and you will see the potential for turning upright rows into

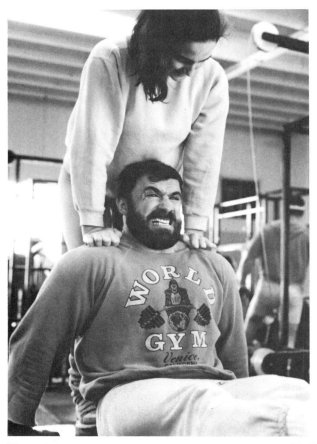
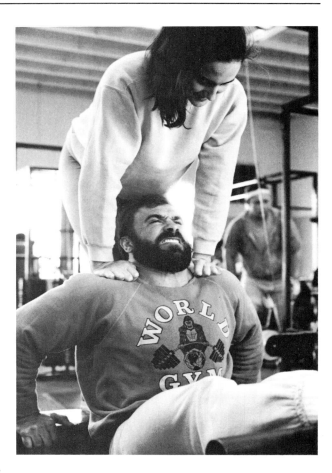

Tricep bench press-ups as demonstrated by Ali Malla.

power cleans; of converting lying triceps extensions into close-grip bench presses; turning sissy squats into regular squats; and going from standing presses into jerk presses. Get the idea? It comes down to this: if you refuse to terminate your set when everyone else terminates their sets, you are involving more muscle fibers in the exercise. When you involve additional muscle fibers you build more muscle. OK?

Most trainers like to use barbells for working their lats, especially in exercises like the bent-over rowing exercise. But don't neglect the use of dumbbells. It may sound crazy, but bent-over rowing with two dumbbells can be very effective. In fact, some people claim they get a superior stretch if they perform the alternate dumbbell row, lifting one hand at a time. Don't laugh until you try it. The same goes for the lateral-raise exercise for the side deltoid. Try to hold two dumbbells and perform the exercise in an alternate-raise fashion. It looks a bit kooky, but many people find they lift in better style and with more weight than when they do the two-arms-together lateral raise. If you're in a rut, give it a try. You've nothing to lose if your present training is not giving you the size you want.

"FEEDER" WORKOUTS— SHORTCUT TO SUCCESS!

In this age of advanced training principles, space-age-technology exercise machines, and scientific food supplements, and when everybody is looking for the "secret," the edge that makes the difference between winning and losing, it is surprising that more people don't know what a "feeder" workout is. This is an effective training principle that is not commonly used, and yet it is one of the best ways to speed muscle growth.

The idea of feeder workouts is not new. In fact, certain enlightened people have been doing feeder workouts for more than 30 years. Maybe longer. Many of the top champions of the last two decades have been using feeder workouts (or a variation thereof) right under our noses.

Just what is a feeder workout and how does it improve your training results? A feeder workout is a light, high-rep, low-set pumping workout done in a separate training session, usually on the day after the regular workout for a muscle group. The purpose of the feeder workout is not to severely work the muscle again or try to tire it out and break down more tissue, but to remove waste products from the muscle (which will alleviate or take away any soreness) and, most important, to nourish the muscle with rich blood. The feeder workout aids in tissue repair, improves blood circulation, increases recovery abil-

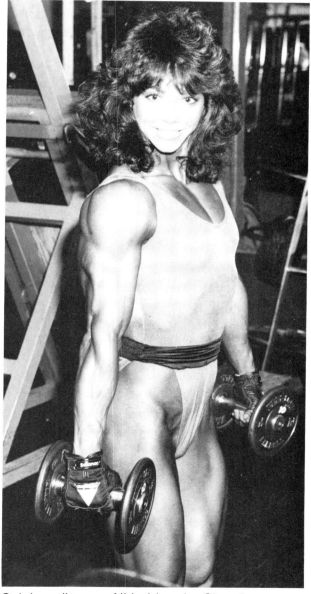

Catch a glimpse of this rising star Clare Furr.

69

ity—and thus lets you respond faster to your training.

Let's examine why this happens.

In bodybuilding and weight training, the pump—getting a lot of blood into the muscle—is of paramount importance. The more blood you can move through a muscle, the more it will respond to the weight training. This is because the more blood a muscle receives, the more nutrients it gets and the more waste products are removed, all of which greatly enhance conditions for growth.

In order for a muscle to grow, it basically needs two things:

1. It must be stimulated to grow via some kind of overload.
2. It must be given the opportunity to grow by being provided with the right conditions for recovery—which **allow** it to grow.

Just because you've done a heavy workout to stimulate growth in a particular muscle group doesn't mean the muscle group will grow if the conditions are not *right* for growth. The stimulation provided by a heavy workout is normally not enough in itself for growth to occur. The muscle must recover and rebuild before the next workout, or it will not grow bigger or stronger.

The recovery ability, then, is as important as the exercise itself. There are many factors involved in promoting recovery ability. Some of these are:

1. Good basic body health.
2. The amount of conditioning and training your body has experienced.
3. Being careful not to overtrain.
4. Allowing for rest, sleep, and recuperation time between training sessions.
5. A good diet that provides plenty of protein and nutrients to repair tissue, build muscle, and keep the body functioning optimally.
6. Good circulation to the muscle.

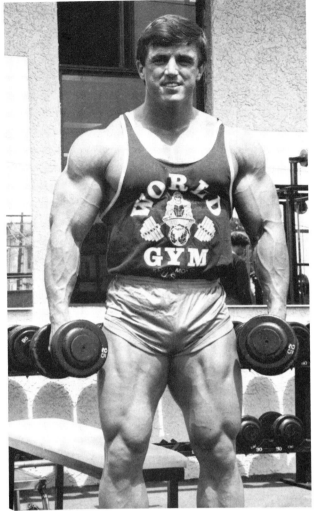

Canada's Andre Maille shows exceptional muscular development.

Since blood is the only means of transporting nutrients to the muscle and removing waste products produced by exercise, it stands to reason that anything that increases blood supply to the muscle will result in faster gains.

High-intensity, heavy workouts give the muscles the stimulation to grow but do little to increase the ability to grow. In fact, such training hinders your recovery ability. The intense workout breaks down a lot of tissue, depletes ribosomes and messenger RNA, and clogs the tissue with lactic acid and other waste products. While these waste products are essential for rebuilding the muscle and replenishing ATP stores (which are essential for energy and muscular contraction), if left in the muscle too long, they can hamper recovery or at least slow the process.

Frequent pumping, on the other hand, greatly increases the ability of muscles to grow by increasing blood circulation and speeding waste removal. This is why your blood vessels grow larger as you train, to facilitate greater blood flow to and from your muscles.

The trouble is, most people either do not remove the waste products and bring in nutrients fast enough to support recovery from their heavy workouts or they remove them too fast by immediately training another muscle group, which flushes the fatigue products out before they have stayed in the muscles long enough to perform their chemical duties.

If pumping is so good, why not just pump all the time? Well, some people can and do. Serge Nubret and Freddie Ortiz found that all they ever had to do to grow big was lots of sets, lots of reps, and pump, pump, pump! These people are genetically superior types who can grow muscle tissue and restore carbohydrate stores, while recovering at the same time. But the large majority of people, because of low hormone levels and poor genetics, can't stimulate muscle growth without high intensity and/or heavy training.

But as I just explained, most people who do *just* heavy training usually won't recover well enough to promote growth. So pumping is needed to feed the muscle and promote recovery. The more you pump, the more your body is able to respond to the stimulus from the heavy training.

Believe it or not, according to researchers, circulation to a muscle can be increased to an amazing 50 times greater than normal! This means that pumping a muscle regularly can also increase recovery ability many, many times above normal (up to 50 times!), depending on the amount of pump achieved.

Most people might try to accomplish both types of training in one workout. At first glance it would appear ideal to do some heavy, high-intensity training to promote growth and then immediately do

some high-rep pumping to the same muscle group to increase blood circulation, but doing so flushes out the waste products before they have a chance to perform their necessary chemical duties. It is best to wait an absolute minimum of 20 minutes before doing any light pumping. If possible, it is best to wait an hour or more. But just to make sure, I suggest you wait until the next day before doing the light feeder workout. This way you know for sure you are not interfering with the functions of the waste products. Why do heavy workouts if you're not going to gain maximally from such workouts?

But, remember, these feeder workouts must be light and should not tax the muscle at all. You want to increase blood circulation to the muscle without tiring it out. One to three sets of 15–30 reps with weights that are about 20–30 percent of your normal load is plenty. If you normally use over 300 pounds in the squat for 20 reps, for your feeder workout you need use only 100–135 pounds. If you use 60-pound dumbbells for dumbbell curls, then 15–20

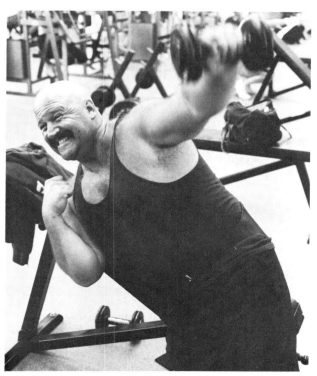

Strongman John Lykes works on a lateral raise movement.

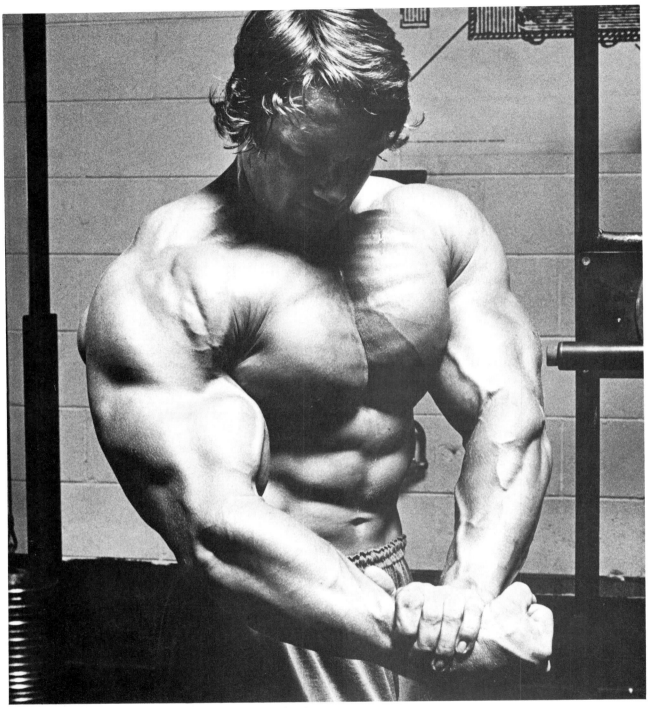

Arnold flexes his incredible chest during a workout.

pounders are all you need for your biceps feeder workout.

I recommend one to three such feeder sets the day after for each muscle group. Most people find that two sets suffice, but the more advanced can do more. So, for example, if you are on a three-day split schedule and working on a push-pull routine, here is how your routine might look:

Day 1: Abs, chest delts, triceps

Day 2: Lats, traps, biceps, forearms

Day 3: Quads, leg biceps, and calves

For your feeder workouts, all you would do is perform your second day's workout with one to three sets from the previous day's routines. On day 2 you would do one to three sets of 15–30 reps each for the abs, delts, and triceps. On day 3 you would do one to three sets of 15–30 reps of lats, traps, biceps, and forearms before starting your leg work. Since day 4 is a rest day, you would sneak in a few extra light feeder sets for your thighs and calves.

It may not be necessary to do feeder sets for all your body parts. *But it is definitely recommended that you do them for your poorly responding or under-par body parts.* You'll have to experiment to see how much you need to do and want to do.

An example of someone who has used feeder workouts is former Mr. Universe Ricky Wayne. Back in the sixties, next to Larry Scott, Ricky had the biggest and best-built arms around. On his days off, Ricky would do three sets of 15 reps of one-arm cable curls and three sets of 15 reps of one-arm tricep pressdowns. It was one of Ricky's secrets.

Currently, Marjo Selin, a top woman bodybuilder from Finland, trains her biceps and triceps on different training days. But on biceps day Marjo adds a couple of light sets for the triceps, and on triceps day she likewise sneaks in a few sets for the biceps. She finds this greatly aids recovery.

Vic Downs, Mohamed Makkawy, Arnold Schwarzenegger, and Franco Columbu all used variations of feeder workouts by sometimes training only one muscle group per training session. In fact, nearly every top star has done some sort of training in which one or two closely related muscle groups are worked heavily and then rested for several hours before other body parts are trained. Whether or not they knew the technical reason for doing this, it seems they instinctively knew it was the right thing to do. Serge Nubret would train a body part for an hour and then sleep for a while, right in the gym, before moving on to a different body part.

A few key points to remember: if you expect to nourish your muscles with the blood you pump in, you had better be eating properly to ensure nutritious, rich blood. When going for maximum growth, Arnold Schwarzenegger advocated 1½–2 grams of protein per pound of body weight. Eat plenty of meat, fish, chicken, eggs, and milk, as well as lots of vegetables, fruits, and some breads. At least one food from each food group, to ensure a balanced diet.

Take your supplements, too. Amino acids have revolutionized bodybuilding. They allow you to get plenty of protein

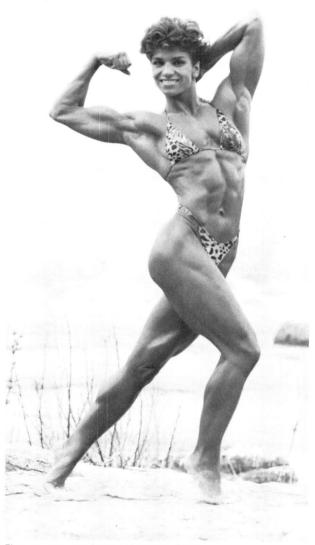

The gorgeous form of Marjo Selin.

without too many fattening calories and with no stomach bloating. They also keep your blood sugar up and keep your body in positive nitrogen balance.

Liver tablets are a good supply of protein, minerals (especially iron), B vitamins, and the energy factor P-450. They also keep blood sugar levels elevated, keep you in positive nitrogen balance, and contain an antiestrogen factor.

A good milk and egg protein will supply you with extra calories and protein if you are trying to gain weight. You should also take a good high-potency vitamin-mineral tablet, extra vitamin C, A, D, and E, plus wheat germ oil for a supply of unsaturated fatty acids.

Give feeder workouts a try. You're sure to see improved results from your training; but bear in mind this is advanced training and should only be used by those who are stuck with more conventional training methods, unable to advance to a new plateau.

WORLD GYM SUPERSTARS— TIPS FROM THE TOP

Just about all the top names in the pro ranks have spent time at World Gym. The impressive building in Venice is affectionately known as the *Home of Bodybuilding's Biggest Stars.* Its best known patrons include my close friends Arnold Schwarzenegger, Franco Columbu, Bob Paris, Lou Ferrigno, Tom Platz, and Frank Zane. All are top pros, and each has carved out a successful career in bodybuilding and show business—including films, television commercial endorsements, and even live legitimate theater. There are of course hundreds more. When out-of-town champions visit Venice one of the places they simply have to train at is my new World Gym establishment at 812 Main St. And, of course, our franchise system, which extends around the globe, has both established and budding stars among its legion of members.

World Gym trainers are among the most knowledgeable in the business. They are winners; their advice on training and diet is worth hearing. Sometimes a few words from a champion bodybuilder can change your progress from *standstill* to tremendous.

ARNOLD SCHWARZENEGGER

I have to admit that even though I have seen Arnold regularly now for over 20 years, he still amazes me. When he first

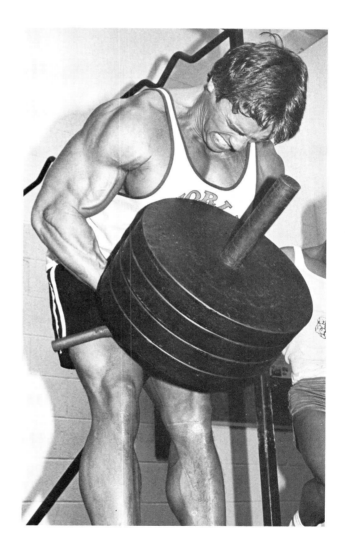

came to my gym he was quite bulky. His chest was just under 60 inches and his arms were over 22. He owed his bulk to hard training and Blair's milk and egg protein, which he gorged on between workouts. He trained like a crazy kid in the late sixties, and his biggest problem came after his workouts when he tried to get into his Volkswagen, which Joe Weider had rented for him as part of their contract. I once made reference to Arnold, about his being slightly less than ripped— but I never had to do it again. When Olympia time came around he trounced the competition again and again. Not only did he have the biggest physique, but he had the most proportionate *and* the most cut physique in the show. During Arnold's winning streak his victory was never in doubt. The question on everyone's mind was who was going to come in second!

"The mind is incredible," Arnold says. "Once you've gained mastery over it, channeling its powers *positively* for your purposes, you can do anything. I mean anything. The secret is to make your mind work for you, not against you. I believe in always being positive, setting up challenges and then going all out for their achievement. You should strive to improve your body a little bit at a time. Don't push the mind excessively; allow it to stay hungry for more success. Beginners, or those getting back into bodybuilding, should start small with an easy program. Time will pass, and each workout you can do more, increasing the weight, sets, and reps to add to the overall intensity."

Actually, Arnold was the first superstar bodybuilder to use the double split schedule. He started it in Europe while working as a gym instructor. Because of his duties he was forced to train from nine to eleven in the morning and then again from seven to nine at night. It worked well for him, although for many this would constitute too much work. When he came to America to train at my gym he continued to split his workouts. Typically he would train from nine to ten-thirty and then again from six to seven-thirty in the evening. Between workouts he would have a light lunch, drink half a gallon of milk and egg protein, gobble down some amino acid tablets, and relax on the beach with

Franco and his ever-growing band of friends.

Arnold experimented with every conceivable type of exercise routine, but one of his favorite systems was the triple-drop (or stripping routine). Typically he would start an exercise, say the barbell curl, and after five or six heavy reps, his training partners would quickly remove two plates; and then after several more reps even more weight would be removed. His last reps would be almost impossible to finish. He felt this was one of the best ways to destroy his muscles in the shortest possible time.

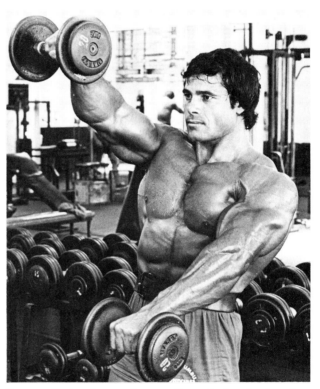

Franco Columbu performs alternate front raises for the front delts.

FRANCO COLUMBU

Back in 1969 Arnold persuaded Joe Weider to fly Franco over from Europe so that they could train together in my gym. Franco turned out to be a powerhouse. After all, he was a successful European powerlifter. In most exercises, because of his short limbs (giving him advantageous

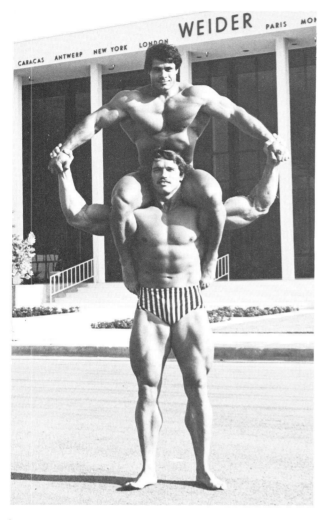

FRANCO COLUMBU'S TRAINING ROUTINE

Monday and Tuesday
Morning (chest, back, stomach)

Bench Presses	5 × 8
Incline Bench Presses	4 × 8
Dips	4 × 12
Flyes	3 × 10
Chins Behind the Neck	5 × 10
Chins Front	5 × 10
T-Bar Rowing	4 × 10
Pulley	4 × 10
Crunches	4 × 25
Bent-Leg Sit-Ups	4 × 25
Lying Side-Leg Raises	4 × 25

Evening (shoulders, calves)

Bent-Over Lateral Raises	4 × 10
Lateral Raises	4 × 10
Presses Behind the Neck	3 × 10
Front Raises	3 × 10
Donkey Raises	7 × 15
Calf Raises	5 × 10

Tuesday and Friday
(arms)

Incline Dumbbell Curls	5 × 10
Triceps Pressdowns	5 × 10
Lying Triceps Extensions	5 × 10
Dumbbell Curls	4 × 10
Sitting Incline Barbell Extensions	5 × 10
Preacher's Bench	4 × 10

Wednesday and Saturday
(thighs, calves, stomach)

Leg Extensions	5 × 20
Leg Curls	4 × 20
Squats	5 × 10
Leg Presses	4 × 20
Donkey Raises	7 × 15
Calf Raises	5 × 10
Crunches	4 × 25
Bent-Leg Raises	4 × 25
Side-Leg Raises	4 × 25

leverage), he used considerably more weight than others outweighing him by 50 pounds, Arnold included. Franco trained at his own slow pace, and he loved the basics—squats, deadlifts, bench press, behind-neck press, and rows. Within three years of giving up strict powerlifting for bodybuilding, Franco became Mr. Universe. What an achievement! Today he runs his own chiropractic clinic and is in constant demand for TV, films, seminars, and guest appearances.

When Franco is asked to recommend a good training routine for an advanced bodybuilder, he points to his successful blitz routine, which was included in his book, *Franco Columbu's Complete Book of Bodybuilding* (Contemporary Books, Chicago). It's similar to the routine he used to win his Olympia titles:

FRANK RICHARDS

He's Britain's comeback man, so named because at the peak of his career he had an accident at work in which he fell more than 30 feet and broke just about every bone in his body. Fourteen operations later he came back to the sport. Frank

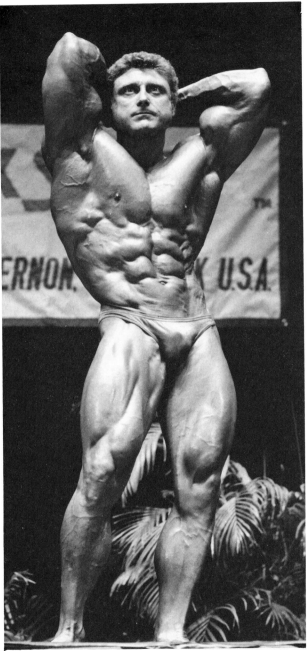

Frank Richard in fine form.

dumbbell presses, cable upright rows, and barbell shrugs.

Frank starts his sets with about 15 reps (he doesn't count them) and then begins adding weight for the next two sets. Usually this enables him to do about 12 reps for the second set and 8 for the third.

Frank is a heavy eater. He consumes an enormous 8,000 calories a day and doesn't get fat. Early in the season he eats four good meals a day. Breakfast consists of porridge, six eggs, a half pound of ham, beans, and pancakes with syrup. For lunch he'll eat half a chicken, a baked potato, cottage cheese, a green salad, and tea or coffee. His third meal is a steak, a baked potato with cheese topping, a half-dozen eggs, and peas. Finally at night before retiring he'll have an omelet with ham and cheese, plus a couple more baked potatoes, topped off with a can of peaches for dessert. His supplements consist of free-form amino acids, liver tabs, mega B-complex capsules, vitamin C (three grams), vitamin E (1,200 IU), three iron tablets, three zincs, three potassium, three megamineral tabs, and about 30 brewer's yeast tablets.

LEE HANEY

Actually, Lee has his own gym in his super home, but when he's in town I'm always pleased to see him training at World's. Lee likes to vary his workouts: "It keeps my muscles off balance, and I find that this is one of the secrets to regular growth."

Lee is one of those people, and there are many, myself included, who believe that twice-a-week training is ideal for overall growth, but because his biceps were under par to the rest of his physique, he decided to experiment and train them three times a week instead of the normal two. And it worked! "Within three or four weeks I began to see my biceps growing like crazy, coming up like a volcano on a virgin plain," Lee said.

Lee also credits his new mental approach. He had always concentrated hard, but he had never actually visualized his

trained with Arnold at my first hard-core gym in Venice.

Today he's still competing and making better progress than ever. His best body parts are his enormous coconut delts. He does three sets of 8–15 reps on the following exercises, twice weekly: seated bent-over laterals, cable bent-over laterals, standing dumbbell lateral raises, Smith machine behind-neck presses, seated

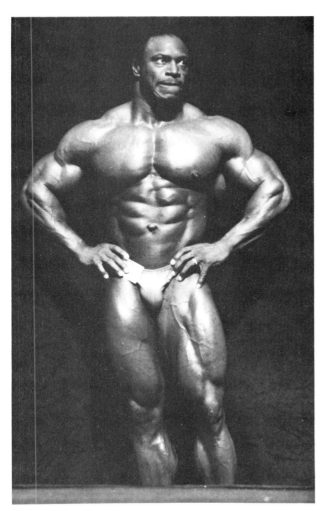

The massive Lee Haney.

MATT MENDENHALL

Matt Mendenhall is undoubtedly one of the stars of the eighties and nineties. He has some of the most enviable genetic gifts of any bodybuilder. Matt started bodybuilding because he broke his arm while pole-vaulting at a high school practice meet: "The pole broke and I fell, missing the pit, to the runway. My arm was broken so badly that I was in a cast for 20 weeks. When I finally got the cast off I spent a whole year in physical therapy, but the movement didn't come back completely until I tried weight training at my doctor's suggestion."

This got him into training with barbells and dumbbells, but he admits he didn't take his training seriously. Today he is a champion and trains using a split cycle schedule: "I work out six days a week; I train chest and biceps on Mondays and Thursdays, back and triceps on Tuesdays and Fridays, and legs and shoulders on Wednesdays and Saturdays." He exercises his abs almost every day. Matt trains his large muscle groups—chest, back, and thighs—using 20–25 sets; for the smaller areas—shoulders, biceps, and triceps—he sticks to no more than 15 sets for each area. "I work the smaller body parts very fast," Matt says, "no more than 45 seconds rest between sets, but for heavier exercises I give myself more time to recover."

Matt is known for his super chest development; the following is one of the routines he follows for that area. He trains his chest twice weekly:

biceps getting bigger. "Once I began 'seeing' a high peak on my biceps," he said, "I began to get that peak. So every night I worked harder and longer in 'seeing' the type of biceps development I wanted. And ultimately it just happened!" Here is a typical week of biceps training by the multi-Mr. Olympia winner:

Monday

Standing Barbell Curls	5 × 8-10
Incline Dumbbell Curls	5 × 6-8
Barbell Preacher Curls	5 × 8-10

Thursday

Standing Dumbbell Curls	5 × 6-8
Barbell Preacher Curls	5 × 8-10
Dumbbell Concentration Curls	5 × 10-12

Saturday

Dumbbell Concentration Curls	5 × 10-12
Cable Curls	5 × 6-8

Incline Dumbbell Press	5 × 6-10
(110 to 120 lb. dumbbells)	
Flat Bench Dumbbell Press	5 × 10
(130-150 lb. dumbbells)	
Pek-Dek Flyes	5 × 10
Cross Bench Dumbbell Pullover	5 × 12
Cable Crossovers	4 × 12

When Matt chooses to bench-press in the off-season he usually hits 450 pounds for several reps. This gives you an idea how amazingly strong he is.

Matt's diet in the off-season is pretty

liberal. He does, however, try to have a high-protein food with every meal: "I'm concerned mainly with keeping my protein intake high, to at least 150–200 grams a day." Twelve weeks before a competition he drops his calories to 1,800 a day, eating mainly fish, turkey, chicken, fresh vegetables, and fruit. Matt is a champion whose ultimate success is written in the stars.

TOM PLATZ

Tom has been a supporter of World Gym for a long time. When he trains, people still stop and stare—and when he trains those unbelievable legs of his, they positively ogle.

When my coauthor, Robert Kennedy, who incidentally helped me greatly with organizing my thoughts for this book, came to town for my new World Gym opening, he sat speechless as Platz trained. "I've seen him train before," Kennedy said, "but he's getting more out of each set than ever before. It's truly amazing. Tom is the hardest-training bodybuilder of all time!" I had to agree with Robert. Platz is indeed a modern-day phenomenon. For example, during his leg extensions, he uses such heavy weights that he has to be strapped to the bench! When he squats he goes into a new dimension. It's like a religion. With hundreds of pounds on his back he squats

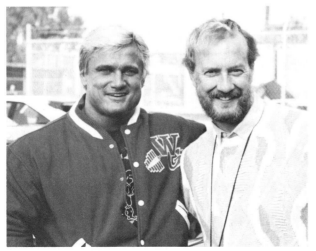

The Golden Eagle with my co-author Bob Kennedy.

deeper than anyone else and squeezes out endless reps. When you think he's done he'll do another 10 reps! It's way beyond anything else I have seen in this crazy world of bodybuilding.

Let's just peek into a typical set of incline curls. Tom will lie back on the bench, set at about a 75-degree angle, which is pretty steep for incline curls, but that's the way he likes it. He locks himself tight against the upright, his legs stretched out straight in front of him. He begins to curl the 70-pound dumbbells one at a time. As the dumbbell reaches his chest he holds it in position and squeezes his biceps, not for a second but for five or six seconds. He does the same with the other arm. He repeats this alternate curling for several more reps, all very strict, until he can do no more. It's the end of the set. But no! It isn't. Tom now slides forward on the bench to afford himself better leverage. Amazingly, without pause, he continues curling—just watching him makes your throat dry. It goes on and on. When is he going to stop? Finally the weights won't budge anymore. It's the end of the set.

But no! It isn't. Tom hangs on to the weights, his arm straight. He tries to curl them. With all his effort . . . he tries. His elbows bend slightly. The dumbbells rise half an inch. It's nothing like a curl, but it is an attempt. The pain is written all over Tom's face. He is trying to curl weights that won't budge. He holds on, refusing to let go. He knows he is benefiting from the effort. Anyone else in the bodybuilding world would have dumped off the weights by now and flopped to the floor exhausted. Finally the set ends.

But no! It doesn't. In a last-ditch effort of crazed fury Tom swings the bells in an exaggerated cheat fashion for a further 8-10 all-out reps. He's throwing the weights up, gasping for air, groaning with pain—reaching out and grabbing all the biceps stimulation and pain he can muster. Finally, in a spasm of temporary exhaustion, he drops the bells. The set has ended.

Yes, it has! Then Tom goes on to perform *seven* more similar sets for his biceps.

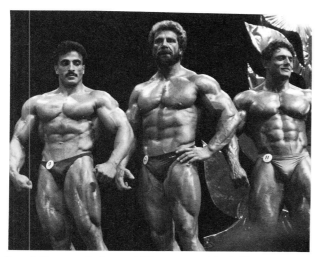

Samir Bannout, Jusup Wilcosz, and Bob Birdsong.

SAMIR BANNOUT

Samir has a great line to his body, and with intelligent training he has improved this markedly. For several years Samir was plagued by a water-retention problem caused by sodium in his body. Frequently he became tense and stressed before a competition, which would cause his body to release large quantities of the hormone aldosterone, which in turn made his body hoard sodium. The sodium then retained excess water, robbing Samir of the needed definition required to win a top competition. Ultimately Samir beat the problem by learning to relax more and by consuming relatively large amounts of sodium up to three days before an event, to suppress the aldosterone output. "I would then go to zero sodium for three days," Samir said, "and the aldosterone release couldn't kick back in, and I was able to free my body of sodium and water. Now I can come into any show ripped to shreds. No one can beat me."

Watching Samir train at my World Gym I have noticed that he is very much an instinctive trainer. He does not work out with the Platz intensity, but he works with a special "feel" for each movement. He knows exactly what part of his body is working. And he carefully tailors each exercise to improve his overall shape and line. There is no guesswork in Samir Bannout's training regime. In his excellent book, *Mr. Olympia's Muscle Mastery* (New American Library), Samir gives us his training philosophy: "Less than optimum mental drive and commitment limit the ultimate intensity of a workout and hence prevent maximum muscular growth. All-out, balls-to-the-wall bodybuilding workouts produce outstanding physiques, and high-intensity workouts are impossible without optimum commitment." That about sums up the man. His physique and mental commitment are bigger than life.

GARY STRYDOM

When this monster of a man first came to California from South Africa it wasn't long before he became a regular at World Gym. Gary is one tough trainer. Take his lower legs, for example. They have to be among the biggest in bodybuilding, yet he still trains them like a madman. He will alter-

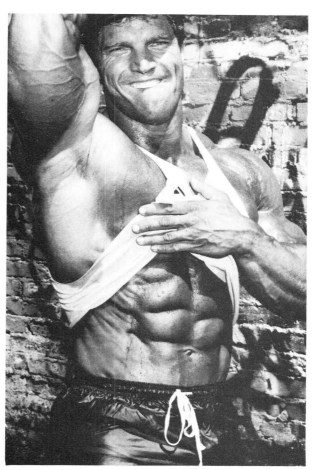

Gary Strydom shows some serious cuts.

nate set after set of seated calves with standing calves until his underpins blow up to over 20 inches. And if his pump isn't satisfactory, he'll go over to the 45-degree leg press machine and perform several sets of complete-range toe raises to make doubly sure the pump arrives. Gary is over six feet tall and has a fast metabolism. He burns up almost everything he eats. In the off-season he has to eat around 6,000 to 8,000 calories a day just to maintain weight. As a competition approaches he cuts back to 4,000 a day, but seldom less.

"I eat every two hours—lots of steamed vegetables and poultry, baked potatoes and boiled fish," Gary says. "I have to thank my wonderful wife, Alyse, for her help with regard to my nutrition. She even went to the trouble of using a computer to work out how my individual characteristic variables would affect my calorie require-

ments. Things like frame size, muscle mass, metabolic rate, fat levels. . . ."

The typical Strydom diet is to eat six times as follows:

Breakfast 7:00 A.M.
5 eggs, all of the whites and 3 yolks
2 slices of whole-wheat toast and bowl of sliced fruit
2 to 3 jars of baby-food fruit for quick-acting carbohydrate energy
Carbohydrate powder
Workout One: 8:30 A.M. to 10:00 A.M.
Midmorning Snack: After Workout
2 steamed chicken breasts, without skins
2 baked potatoes, dry
Fruit juice or sparkling water
Workout Two: 11:30 A.M. to 1:30 P.M.
Lunch: After Workout
Tuna salad, tossed with lettuce, tomatoes, vegetables, and sprouts—no dressing except for a little vinegar
1 slice whole-wheat bread
Orange juice
Afternoon Snack: 5:00 P.M.
1 chicken or tuna sandwich
Piece of fruit
Protein Drink
Dinner: 7:00 P.M.
Steak
Baked potato, dry
Steamed vegetables
Bedtime Snack: 10:00 P.M.
Bowl of oatmeal with milk and fruit

IRVIN "ZABO" KOZEWSKI

Now in his 60s, Zabo looks tremendous. As Gene Mozee says, "Zabo looks like he's caught in a time warp that has kept him at 35 years of age." As a teenager Zabo had to serve in the Army during World War II, and while on duty in the Pacific he contracted malaria. But two years later, after resuming his training, he had the Mr. New Jersey title under his belt. In 1950 he won the best abdominals at both the Junior and the Senior AAU Mr. America and then for 20-plus years after that he won more than 100 best abs awards, several dozen most-muscular titles, and two dozen physique contests. In 1972, at the age of 48,

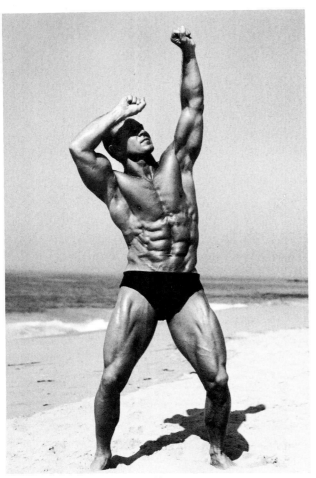

Zabo Kozewski flexes for the camera.

Zabo astounded the bodybuilding fraternity by winning the "world's most muscular man" title in the IFBB Mr. World competition. He beat out athletes less than half his age, but he was most proud of the fact that he did it naturally. "Most of the other competitors were on steriods," he says. "I wasn't, but I still took the Most-Muscular Award. That was my greatest accomplishment."

In 1950, along with Dick Dubois and Dom Juliano, Zabo moved west. That was when I first met him and he trained at my gym. What a gang we were on Muscle Beach. There was Steve Reeves, Harry Schwartz, Chuck Gray, George Eiferman, John Farbotnik, Earle Liederman, Eric Pedderson, Armand Tanny, Roy Hilligen, Dick Dubois, and of course Zabo himself.

How did Irvin Kozewski keep his abdominals so supercut and built at the same time? His formula was simple: he trained his abs six days a week and performed a thousand incline sit-ups and a thousand bench leg raises every workout. Today he does 500 Roman chair sit-ups and 500 bent-knee leg raises three times a week.

"We all enjoyed ourselves greatly in those days," Zabo says. "Bodybuilders were a close-knit group because we were considered weird, so we all hung out together. We were almost outcasts. Today we are just people who train. Heck, there are another 30 million out there now."

Zabo has been one of the World Gym directors for a long time. He's helped me run the gym for almost 30 years. He's still down-to-earth, trains hard, and allows no distractions. "I don't talk to others when I'm training," he says. "Talk never built muscles, so why talk when you should be concentrating one hundred percent on your training?" Makes sense to me.

ED GIULIANI

Here's another guy I can rely on to take care of the gym if I'm out of town or busy with one of my projects. Eddie is originally from New York and has won a variety of titles, including Mr. Western America, Mr. Eastern America, and class wins in the Mr. America and Mr. U.S.A. competitions. His main contribution to the gym is his light-hearted good nature. His spirits are always high, and that's good all around. Like Zabo, Eddie has good abdominal development, and in fact he trains similarly to Zabo in that he prefers high reps with little resistance to low reps with added weights. Typically, Eddie will perform Roman chair sit-ups by the clock (20 minutes nonstop). This translates to around 500–600 reps for the upper abdominals. Then he will perform lying kickouts for the lower abs for 15 minutes—about 500 reps. Eddie is adamant about doing abs at the end of his workout. He says he feels the burn more then because much of his food has been metabolized from the earlier training.

Any time, any day, you're likely to see Eddie drive up to World's in his new Corvette. Take a look at his body. He doesn't enter shows anymore, but he's never out of shape. And besides . . . he keeps me smiling.

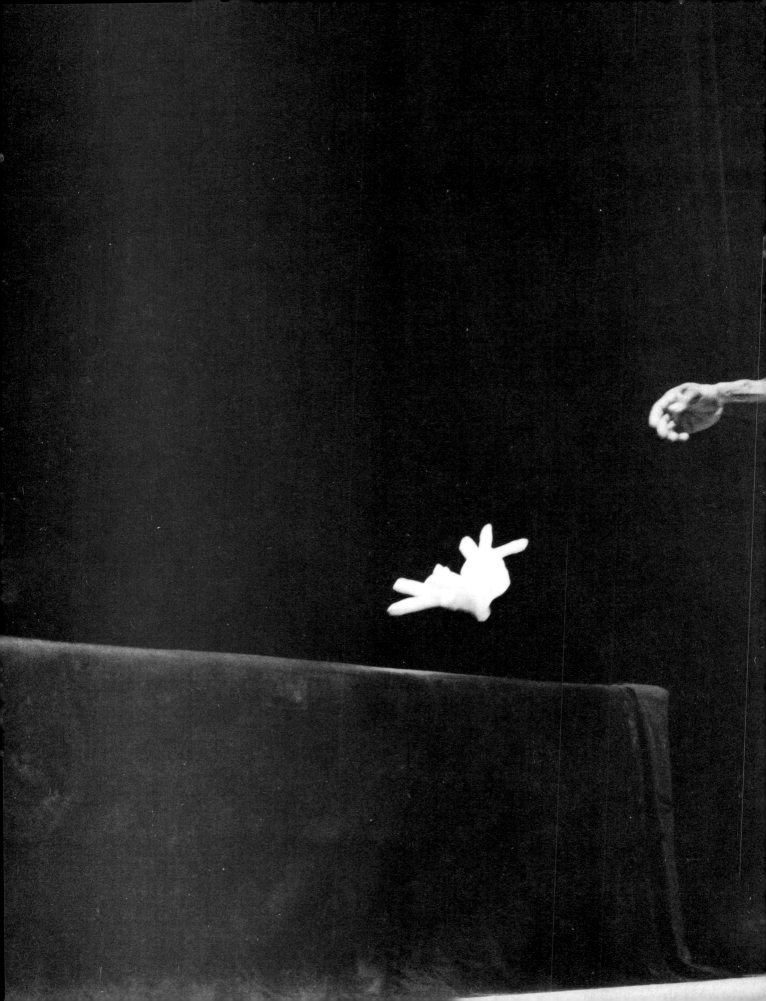

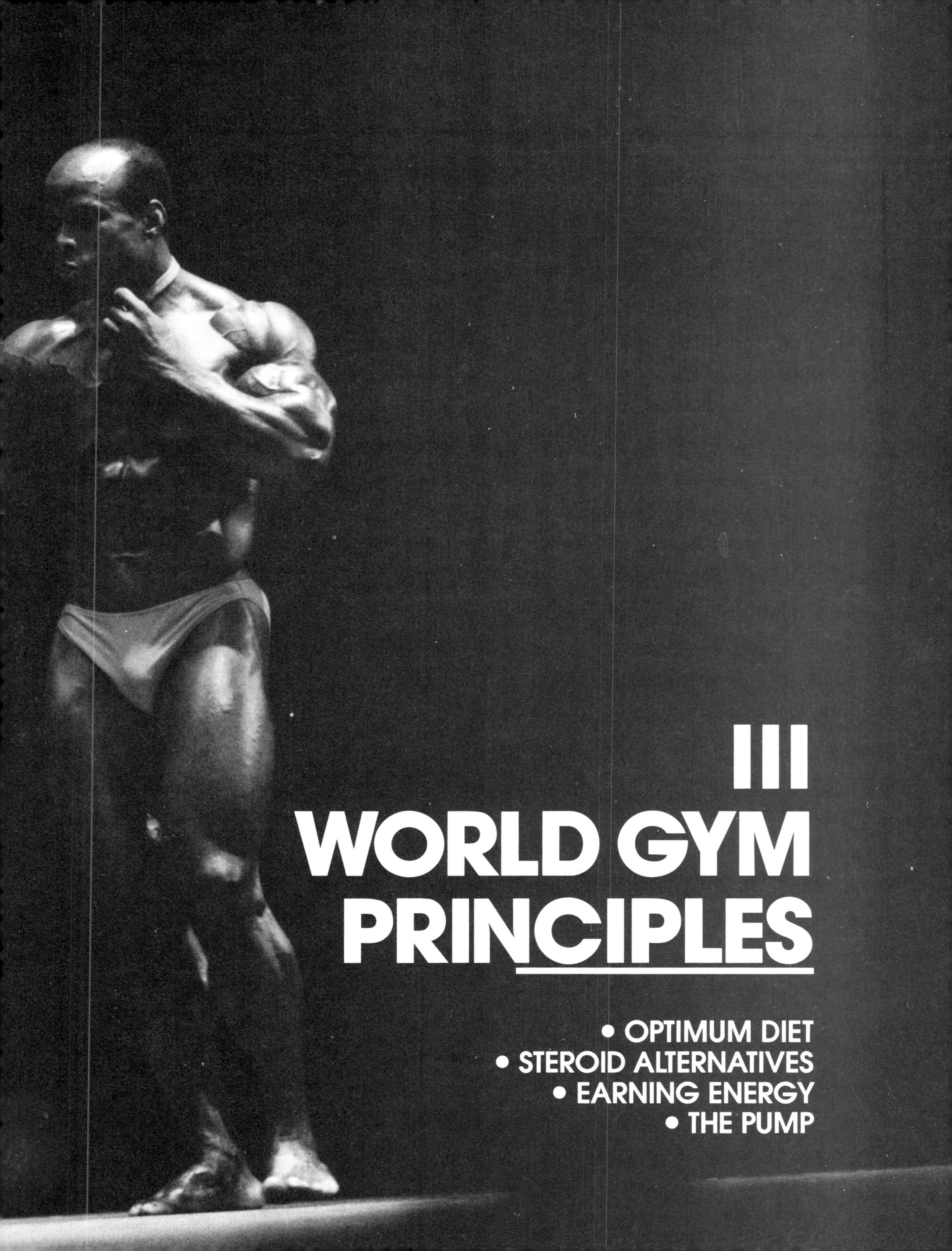

III
WORLD GYM
PRINCIPLES

- OPTIMUM DIET
- STEROID ALTERNATIVES
- EARNING ENERGY
- THE PUMP

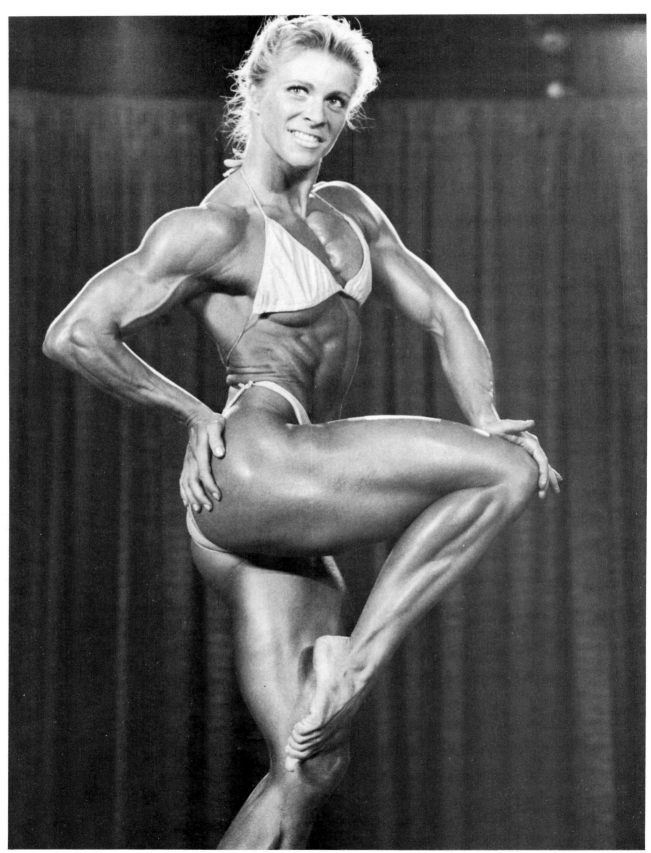

The sensational newcomer, Anja Langer from West Germany.

OPTIMUM DIET—NUTRITION FOR RESULTS

Yes, you can get by on an average diet, which inevitably contains both junk food and desirable foods, but you will not enjoy maximum gains in size, muscularity, or strength. It is only when you follow an optimum diet that you approach one hundred percent of your achievable potential.

Germany's female sensation Anja Langer says: "The food you eat can make or break you as a bodybuilder. Diet is at least half of the ratio. Training know-how is the other half."

Modern scientific studies have verified this premise. Without optimum nutrition you don't have a chance of becoming a champion bodybuilder.

Michael Colgan, Ph.D., designed an individual study to test the relationship between diet and performance. Because it was easier to measure, he chose Olympia lifters to verify the importance of quality nutrition. In one study, his group designed individual diets and supplements for two experienced weight lifters, then measured their gains against that of two others, who were already careful of their diets but unknowingly received placebo (sugar pill) supplements. Pairs trained similarly. Over a three-month period the supplemented lifters gained four to eight percent, while the placebo athletes gained only two per-

cent. In the Olympic lifts, the improvement translated into a total gain of 35 pounds, a significant increase for experienced lifters.

To follow through scientifically, the placebo pair was then also put on the controlled diets and supplements, and within four months they had showed an overall improvement of five percent. So you can conclude that you can gain without optimum nutrition, but you can make better progress with a better diet that includes supplements.

A successful bodybuilding career depends on the proper nutrients to assist the development of muscle, and to help you remain strong and healthy. Basically you should make an effort to avoid junk foods such as potato chips, gravies, cream, jam, canned fruit, pastry, cookies, shortening, candy, chocolate, jelly, soft drinks, vegetable oil, processed cheese, regular breakfast cereals, salad dressings, canned soup, ketchup, ice cream, crackers, and virtually all prepackaged variety store specials.

Your diet should be based on fresh, wholesome foods selected from the basic food groups—otherwise known as the balanced diet. The best way to prepare your food is to keep it as much as possible in its natural state. When you do cook food try to poach, broil, or steam it. Forget about deep frying in heavy fat or using butter, lard, or margarine. Modern science, although it concludes that some dietary fat is necessary, considers the ingredient to be public enemy number one, with sugar and salt tied in the runner-up position.

Good nutrition is vital because it is directly involved in the musclebuilding process. If you eat junk long enough, you will start to look like junk—gray skin, dried-out hair, drooping, dull eyes, scaly skin, etc. Eat fresh, wholesome foods and your complexion will become fresher, your hair will have luster, your eyes will sparkle, and your skin will have a satin-like tone.

Good nutrition for those who want to gain muscle weight quickly can be summed up in a sentence: eat a balanced diet plus a quart of milk a day. A balanced diet means daily portions of each of the following basic food groups.

PROTEIN

Despite being downgraded in importance recently, protein is still the number one food for bodybuilders. You should have a high-protein item with each meal, three to six times a day. Protein is mainly found in meat, fish, poultry, and eggs. Organ meats such as heart, liver, and kidneys are excellent sources. They also provide iron, B vitamins, and certain minerals. Dried beans, nuts, peas, and other legumes are good vegetable sources of protein.

MILK AND MILK PRODUCTS

Milk provides protein, but it is also extremely useful to the bodybuilder in that it is almost the perfect food. All mammals double and triple their body weights on milk alone, and it is a wonderful source of calcium (for bone building), too. Cheeses and yogurts, of course, are products made from milk.

VEGETABLES AND FRUITS

You can't remain healthy without these. They provide vitamins A and C and fiber, and are subdivided into three groups. You should make it a rule as an aspiring body-

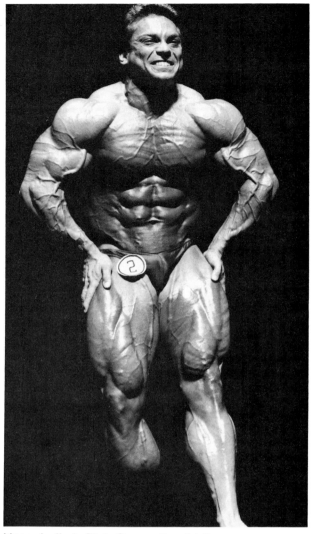

Vascularity is Rich Gaspari's middle name.

builder to have four servings from this category daily.

Group 1

Includes foods rich in vitamin C, such as oranges, lemons, tangerines, cantaloupe, papaya, and strawberries; and such vegetables as broccoli, peppers, Brussels sprouts, cabbage, potatoes, and cauliflower.

Group 2

Includes foods rich in vitamin A: dark, leafy greens such as spinach, beet, collards, and mustard greens; and yellow fruits and vegetables such as squash, carrots, yams, apricots, and peaches.

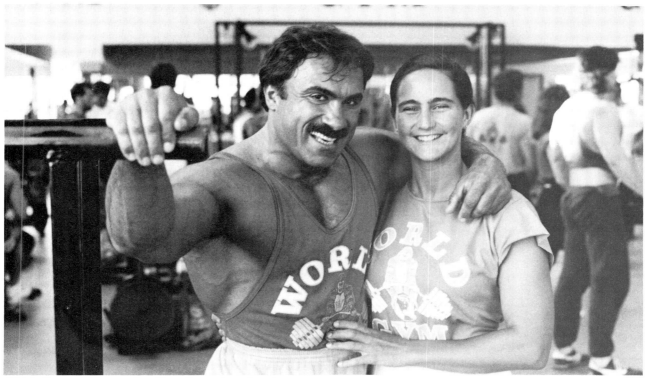

Ali Malla and Shawn Stouffer after a tough set.

Group 3

Includes most other vegetables and fruits, such as lettuce, zucchini, corn, radishes, cucumbers, eggplant, peas, turnips, apples, cherries, bananas, berries, and pears.

GRAIN AND GRAIN PRODUCTS

Includes foods such as whole-wheat bread, whole-grain cereals, etc. These natural, unprocessed grains provide more minerals than so-called "enriched" breads and commercial cereals. They also provide thiamine, niacin, riboflavin, iron, zinc, and phosphorus. Active bodybuilders need at least three servings of grain products daily.

WATER

It is imperative that you drink fresh, clean water every day. Most of our body is made up of water. The president of the United States and the queen of England are made up of two-thirds plain water. Your bones are only one-quarter water, but your muscles (and your brain) are three-quarters water. There is no doubt that plain water is the most important nutrient in your body, even though it has no caloric value. You can survive months without food but only 12 days (at the most) without water. Actually, athletes and bodybuilders in heavy training can lose up to five or more quarts of water in a day. Even a small shortage of water can disrupt your performance and biochemistry. For example, bodybuilders who limit their water intake as a competition approaches invariably lose strength. Dehydrate a muscle by only three percent and you lose ten percent of contractile strength. Maintaining your water intake is the single most important aspect of top training performance.

COMPLEX CARBOHYDRATES

There are simple and complex carbohydrates. Simple carbs are found in sugar, honey, juice, soft drinks, candies, chocolate, etc. Complex carbs are goodies such as brown rice, whole barley, whole rye, wild rice, whole corn, pearl millet, whole wheat, rolled oats, whole buckwheat—and all contain less than five percent fat!

Keep away from too many simple carbohydrates. They disrupt fat metabolism and raise both cholesterol and triglyceride levels. Eat plenty of grains, vegetables, and fruit.

FAT

Bad news all around. Make a strong effort to keep your fat intake low. Check the labels on what you eat. Junk foods like Big Macs, Whoppers, Wendy's Triple Cheeseburgers, Jack in the Box's Bacon and Cheeseburger Supreme are all heavy in fat content. Enough to grease down Lee Haney's back!

Does a high-fat diet influence your cholesterol levels? Actually, cholesterol is not fat; it is a steroid alcohol. Among foods with the highest cholesterol content are butter, egg yolks, hamburger, and liver. As a bodybuilder you should endeavor to keep your cholesterol and blood pressure levels down (your blood pressure should be below 120/80). How can you do this? By eating fewer dairy products (eat low-fat cheese, milk, and milk products, and only have one egg yolk for every three eggs) and by reducing stress factors. Increase your consumption of fish oils and high fiber foods such as whole grains, lentils, mixed beans, steamed vegetables, carrots, cauliflower, pears, bananas, apples, oranges, figs, and prunes.

SUGAR AND SALT

More bad news! The U.S. National Research Council reports that North Americans eat 20 times the salt required for good health. Much of this is found in fast foods, and in processed and canned foods. Check the labels again and keep your salt intake down to one gram a day.

As for sugar, the simple carbohydrate mentioned earlier, it's both harmful and hard to avoid. It's everywhere from bread to baby food, from frozen turkeys to cook-

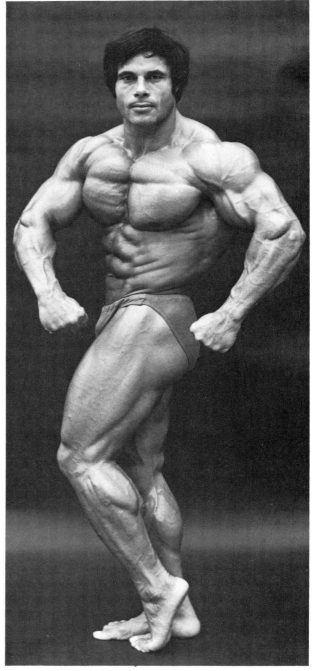

Franco shows incredible muscularity.

ies. As a bodybuilder you had better stick to unprocessed fresh foods in which nature balances out the sugar nicely when you follow a varied diet. Far better, incidentally, to have an apple than apple juice, or a grapefruit than grapefruit juice. Some juices are higher in sugar than regular Coke.

SUPPLEMENTS

Should you supplement your diet? If you want to make optimum gains, the answer must be a resounding yes!

A one-a-day-type vitamin-mineral pill is always a wise investment for the hard-core bodybuilder. It ensures that your training efforts won't be in vain, since vitamin and mineral deficiencies, however unlikely, can hinder progress and even jeopardize overall health.

At one time supplements were not necessary for optimum performance or health, but today we are in a situation of devitalized food, unclean water supplies, frightful canning, freezing, processing, milling and refining procedures, and unnatural livestock raising and breeding. Drying meat, for example, can destroy up to 50 percent of its vitamins and minerals. Commercial baking, using chemical leavening, can destroy more than 90 percent. Do serious bodybuilders need to supplement? You'd better believe it!

STEROID ALTERNATIVES—
NATURAL TRAINING

I'm not going to deny that steroids build more size. As an artificial derivative of the male hormone testosterone they serve to help the body hold more water in the muscle and utilize protein more efficiently. This results in added size and added strength. The trouble with steroids—apart from their obvious side effects such as causing nosebleeds, increased aggressiveness, headaches, bitch-tits, and baldness—is that they can also accelerate heart disease, diabetes, and prostate cancer, and cause severe liver problems later in life. If taken long enough, they will weaken your immune system and will certainly age you prematurely.

Women who take steroids are risking all kinds of horror-story side effects. Increased body hair, deeper voice, and loss of breasts are among the known effects. The unknown is just what heavy prolonged use of steroids by women will produce. Only time will tell what other effects there might be, but you can be sure it won't be good news.

Have you noticed how bodybuilders are tearing their muscles nowadays? This seldom happened in my day, even though we trained hard with forced reps and negatives. Some of the injuries bodybuilders experience are major muscle tears (usually the biceps, triceps, or pectorals). Many

Bob Paris looking serious during the Mr. Olympia competition.

are caused directly by steroid abuse. The drugs increase the strength of the muscle but not of the tendons and ligaments; therefore tears and strains occur more easily.

I don't like the thought of steroid use, even though I know that most of the pros use steroids before competitions. I have heard the old arguments about steroid *use* as opposed to *abuse*. I don't buy it. The parking lot at World Gym is not littered with hypodermic syringes, but over the years I have kicked the odd prescription bottle across the adjoining pavement.

As I see it, steroids make everything grow except the bones. Therefore the physique is seldom improved because the skeletal frame becomes overcrowded with muscle mass. The waistline grows enormously, especially if a bodybuilder has wide hips. . . . I will agree that the hardness factor is relevant and that steroids help this, but so often the user gets hooked and ends up taking steroids for long periods, without giving the body sufficient rest between cycles. The bloated look creeps in and once achieved is seldom lost. A steroid-built body is typified by bunched-up, narrow shoulders, huge drooping pecs, oversized thighs, and a complete inability to pose properly. I've been in the game more than 50 years . . . . It's not a pretty sight!

FREE-FORM AMINO ACIDS

So what are the alternatives? The bodybuilding community was hit by a sudden gust of excitement in the early eighties when Durk Pearson and Sandy Shaw, the authors of *Life Extension: A Practical Scientific Approach* (Warner Books), released the scientific news that growth hormone can be controlled to a certain extent by exercise habits and by supplementation of certain amino acids. They wrote: "There are several nutrients and prescription drugs which cause GH [growth hormone] release." This sounded too good to be true. The next sentence, however, elaborated: "These include the amino acids

arginine and ornithine and the prescription drugs L-dopa (another amino acid), bromocriptine (Parlodel® by Sandoz) and vasopressin (Diapid® by Sandoz, a nasal spray)." In one study by the *Life Extension* authors, one-half gram a day of L-dopa increased the growth hormone output of men in their sixties (who were not suffering from Parkinson's disease) back up to near typical young adult levels.

So the Eagle had landed. Amino acids could trigger the body's mechanism to release more growth hormone. This was it. Every ambitious bodybuilder alive, fed up with the steroid scene, had to have arginine and ornithine. And the results were promising. Pearson and Shaw ran further tests, and their findings proved scientifically conclusive. Large amounts (10 grams or more) of arginine and ornithine injected into human beings *will* trigger the release of human growth hormone (HGH). What followed was a surge of products that contained these amino acids, but in too small dosages to produce noticeable results.

When taking free-form amino acids it is a good idea to start with low dosages and build up slowly. This maximizes their effect without upsetting or shocking the system. Frank Zane writes in *Zane Nutrition* (Simon and Schuster): "When you consider that all the animal proteins come packaged in fat, it makes sense to use amino acids in free form, and eat smaller amounts of animal proteins if you want to keep calories to a minimum."

Zane is the world's number one bodybuilding advocate of free-form amino acids. According to him and his beautiful wife, Christine, a successful bodybuilder in her own right, amino acid supplementation improves feelings of well-being; provides more energy, alertness, and stamina; and increases fat loss, recuperation speed, sex drive, muscle hardness—and more muscle growth! Amino acids provide the nitrogen your muscle cells need for growth, and without additional calories.

Amino acid pills should be swallowed with water or vegetable juice, never taken

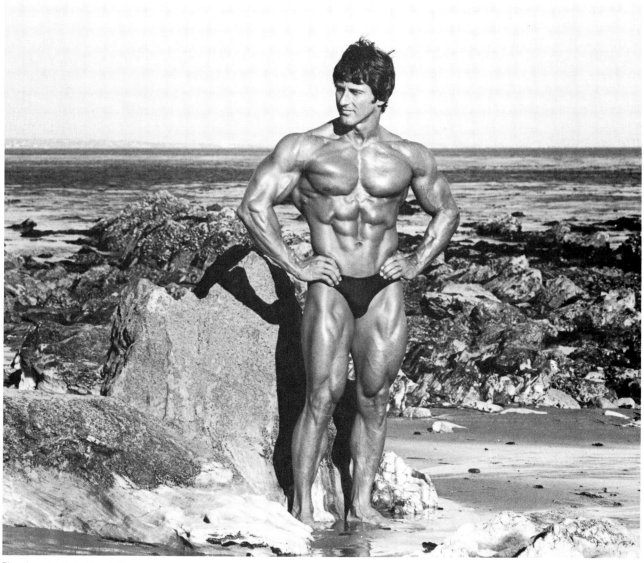

The immortal Frank Zane.

with meals or milk, both of which can hinder absorption by coating the stomach. Add a B-complex vitamin supplement, especially B_6, and a one-a-day multivitamin-mineral tablet.

Having praised amino acid supplementation to the skies, with my fingers crossed that those heavy drug takers will now reduce their dependence on steroids, let me caution you that a few people have congenital amino acid metabolism disorders; therefore I recommend that before going on to any supplemental program you first review your medical history with your doctor or qualified clinical nutritionist. Of course, not all doctors are "up" on

modern nutrition, so if possible seek out an expert who is at least sympathetic to your desire for optimum nutrition.

NATURAL BALANCE

Year after year the confusion reigns. Do bodybuilders require more protein than other athletes or everyday people? Frederick Hatfield, an accomplished author and a man with vast knowledge of nutrition, points to a study done to determine protein requirements among Polish weight lifters. Many were found to be in negative nitrogen balance (using up more protein than they were ingesting) despite their higher than normal protein consumption. The scientific conclusion was that intense weight training greatly increases protein requirements for weight lifters and body-builders.

The answer, then, is to eat small high-protein meals throughout the day. And if you can't find time, supplement your food intake with desiccated-liver pills, or milk and egg protein mixes. (Eggs contain the highest quality protein known; milk runs a close second.)

Natural training can be the most productive type of training because you have time to plan where and how your muscles are built. It is unlikely that you will get stretch marks, bloat out, or bunch up your muscles. You will have more constant energy levels, less breathlessness, and fewer virility fade-outs.

How does natural training differ from training while on steroids? Well, natural training means you will have to train in a more concentrated manner. Every set must count. Recuperation is slightly slower, as is your lasting power. Workouts should be of a good intensity, yet not so demanding as to throw off your recovery periods. For example, if you rely on a 48-hour recovery period for a muscle group,

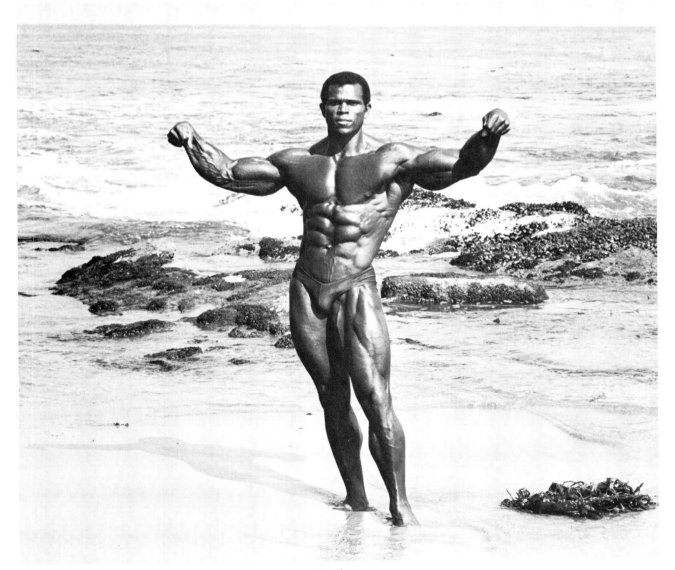

France's Serge Nubret personifies symmetrical proportion.

but you work that area so hard and long that it requires 72 hours to heal, you will be wasting your time training it again after only 48 hours. You'll lose size rather than gain.

When you train *without* steroids, a practice I wholeheartedly recommend, you have to fine-tune your workouts and your diet. Never try to gain or lose more than a pound or two a week. Keep an eye on your calorie intake. Remember bodybuilding photographer John Balik's immortal words: "You can't flex fat!" Fine-tuning means doing the right exercises to build and shape your body correctly. Never perform any exercise unless you are sure what part of your body it is working—and then only if you really need to build that area. *Contrary to popular belief, bodybuilding is not a matter of building every muscle to the max.* This is ridiculous! All of us have areas that build up faster than others, and if we just trained for overall size most of us would be out of proportion. Imagine if Jeff King trained his legs and neck for 20 sets each. Or if Tom Platz squatted heavily twice a week (instead of the one high-rep set of squats a month he does today). No, we have to be discriminating in how we train, and that means our muscles must be built in the right places and in correct proportion to one another for an overall balanced look.

That's where the steroid freaks go wrong. They go for muscle wherever it comes. And they rob their bodies of individuality. Heavy steroid takers all look the same. Bunched up and bloated. *They have thrown away the individuality and natural shape of their bodies, traded it in for primobolan bloat!* Many steroid takers are careless about their diets. Frequently they eat anything and everything—and almost get away with it. A nonsteroid bodybuilder must tailor his or her food intake more carefully. You cannot overload on calories in the hope of building lean mass. You have to add calories slowly, and be prepared to backtrack if you start gaining flab.

As for sets and reps, the natural trainer will not be able to gain from mammoth daily (or twice daily) workouts that some drug takers thrive on. Reps and sets must fall into the moderate range. Typically, reps should fall between eight and twelve. The number of sets should be around four or five, and you should seldom perform more than twelve sets per body part. Train each muscle group two or three times a week. There are, however, exceptions. *Never* cast my words of advice in stone. I'm old and wise enough to know that rules are made to be broken. And frequently are—with a good measure of success.

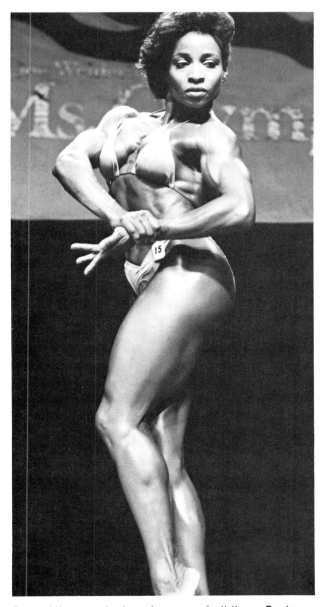

One of the greatest performers of all time, Carla Dunlap.

EARNING ENERGY—LITTLE LEAKS SINK BIG SHIPS

Way back in 1938 in Great Britain thousands of middle-aged men were passing their lives away lazily in noncommital lounging. They were in what could only be described as a recess from living. Life was frequently drab and uneventful—to all extents over. There was little interest, little to do. Until . . . Herr Adolf Hitler marched into Poland.

These same energy-drained beings soon became an active part of Britain's war machine. They joined the armed forces or the home guard. Suddenly they had energy plus, even though at times rations were sparse; frequently they would get only one egg a week; and sleep was limited to the few hours between air raids.

The soldiers trained for combat and fought by land, sea, and air. And the home guard made Britain impregnable. Farmers covered every field with any obstacle they could find to prevent enemy planes from landing on British soil. Ordinary people, anxious to help, rotated long hours of duty standing on top of city buildings with sacks of sand to put out any fires started by air raids. Factory workers toiled in cellars for 18-hour shifts, making arms and ammunition for a meager wage.

These people, once bereft of energy and enthusiasm, had been rejuvenated beyond belief. They had purpose, and it was this inspiration that gave them a new-found zest.

Today in North America and other Westernized countries, millions of people are suffering from an energy crisis. They are locked into apathy and a devitalized existence. And there is no war to wake them up.

Do you lack energy? Do you envy the person who wakes up at the crack of dawn, who is on the go all day and ready for more at night?

Actually, energy levels are partly inherited, but many who suffer from constant tiredness owe the condition to poor lifestyle habits.

Eating Patterns

When do you eat? Most North Americans have coffee and toast for breakfast, a green salad for lunch, more coffee and a heavy-on-the-meat binge meal in the evening. This type of diet is hard on the body and draining on stamina. It robs you of calories in the daytime, when you need them, and provides them plentifully at night, when you don't. This type of eating can cause midafternoon blahs and can sneak on unwanted pounds, since we burn fewer pounds when we sleep. Extra fat on our bodies means less energy—we have to carry fat, whereas pure muscle carries us.

When you eat too few calories in the morning or at lunch, the body frequently lowers its basal metabolic rate to preserve energy. This in itself results in lack of vitality.

Provide calories evenly and generously during the morning and early afternoon. In this way you will raise your metabolic rate and help stave off evening overloads. Eat four or five times a day. No huge meals—ever.

Watch what you eat. Time and time again, I see promising bodybuilders downing junk food a cat wouldn't touch. Eating poor-quality food sabotages your workout efforts. It slows up your rate of recuperation, and the nutrients you need to build that extra muscle are missing from junk foods. But it gets worse. Junk foods are invariably high in sugar and salt. Sugars

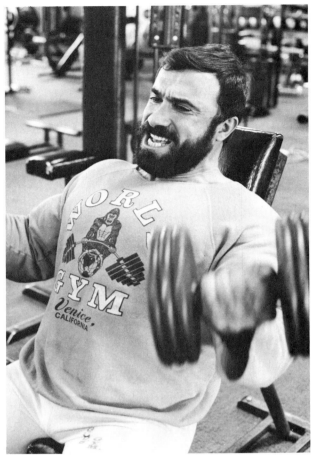

Bearded Ali Malla performs the two-handed dumbbell curl.

contain "empty" calories that can only contribute to adding fat. And if anything can make a potentially well-muscled body look lousy, it's fat. It fills in the spaces between muscles, robbing you of separation and destroying body definition, and killing off any chance you have of looking shapely and attractive. Salt in the amounts you obtain in fast foods and other junk products is positively dangerous. Not only does it lead to hypertension but it can lead to a bloated, unhealthy appearance. Let's drop this junk food talk once and for all. Just take my word for it. I've been hanging around this mudball for a few years now, so listen to me. Cut the junk food! Stick to wholesome fruits, lean meats, fish, vegetables, and grains. Take an apple instead of a sugar-loaded soft drink. Always make sure your meals contain both carbohydrates and protein.

Carbs eaten alone make it easier for the amino acid tryptophan to get out of the bloodstream and into the brain cells, causing drowsiness—fine at bedtime but not when you are at work during the day. When you take protein with your carbs other amino acids compete with tryptophan to get into the brain. In short, emphasize starches and fruits at night for a good sound sleep, but for zest by day add proteins such as milk to your whole-grain cereal, and turkey or fish to your lunchtime salad.

SMOKING

Look at a heavy smoker and observe the shortened stride, the bent back, the concave chest, the gray face, the bloodshot eyes, the trembling hands, the slurred speech, the slow mind, and the complete lack of God-given vitality and zest.

Smoking, even moderately, hardens your blood vessels, cuts your wind, causes cancer and coronary thrombosis, and robs you of the joy of physical movement.

Doctors are quite clear about smoking being bad for your health, but what seems to be coming out of the woodwork now is that smoking and heavy exercise can be twice as bad as smoking by itself. "It's like putting your foot on the gas and the brake at the same time," says Dr. Andrew Pipe, an expert on exercise and smoking at Ottawa's Civic Hospital. Evidence shows that weight lifters and weight trainers have a lot to worry about if they smoke. Lifting weights greatly increases blood pressure and the chance for bursting arteries. Smoking also boosts blood pressure and can mean "double jeopardy," Pipe says, "because the vessels and arteries lose elasticity and harden."

For as long as I remember, tobacco companies have maintained there is no link between smoking and health problems, or physical performance. I wonder how many packs a day their directors smoke?

For the last 40 years we have had plenty of evidence that smoking leads to heart disease and cancer and about a million other complications.

More recently, scientists have studied smoking's short-term effects—among them decreased ability to move necessary oxygen to the muscles. They are coming to the conclusion that smokers should be careful about high-intensity exercise. Be warned!

ALCOHOL

Bring on the booze! I guess you could call Los Angeles the drinking capital of the world. We probably have more alcoholics per square mile than anywhere else on earth. (We also have more gyms and bodybuilders per square mile, so L.A.'s demographics are not all bad.)

I've pleaded with some people to give up booze, but they were gripped by alcohol so strongly that in most cases I was unsuccessful. Occasionally my words got through and I saved a soul or two.

Drinking has its place. Indeed, science tells us that one or two drinks a day are actually good for us. But then they caution that three or more a day can pickle our

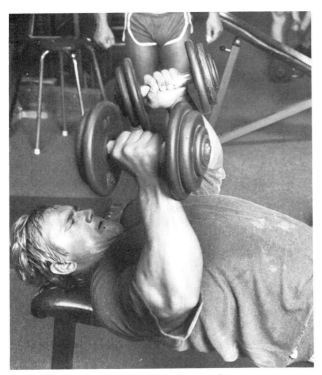

Tom Platz performs a set of incline flyes.

livers, harden our arteries, and give us heart attacks. There seems to be a fine line here. I'll reserve my comments on moderate drinking. What is most definitely wrong is excessive drinking. And excessive *regular* drinking will not only kill your pump, it will kill you.

One fellow in my gym, a most delightful, well-loved man with a physique straight out of the Grecian mold, got caught up with vodka and orange juice. Soon it became plain vodka. And it wasn't long after that when he would dispense with the glass and just drink himself into a stupor straight from the bottle—and on a daily basis. It broke my heart!

Remember that alcohol is a relaxant and a depressant. A single beer or glass of liquor at lunchtime can drain you of energy for the rest of the afternoon. The exact effects depend on your individual metabolism, but for most people a midday drink rules out a high-energy afternoon. If your energy levels are already in the habit of taking a nosedive, just one glass of wine can lead to a near comatose condition.

R&R (REST AND RECUPERATION)

Along with nutrition, rest and sleep help you recover between workouts. Going to bed late and not getting enough sleep will harm your progress. More than that, it will *prevent* your progress. Over the years at World Gym I have known some party animals. I must give them their due. They still keep tossing iron, but they have to party, too. I hear the stories of the booze, the jokes, the gals, and the foot-long cigars. They come into the gym with eyes more bloodshot than a Florida orange. Yes, they keep training—most of the time. But they *never* get better. And that's what bodybuilding is all about: getting better and better. It's built into the very nature of barbell training. Weights are designed so that extra poundage can be added every week or every month. It's the only way to improve the size, shape, and strength of your body. But you need a relaxed hassle-free lifestyle to make it work.

We all have an ideal amount of time we should sleep. For most of us this amounts to 7-9 per night. Some can do well on only six hours of sleep, while a few need as much as ten hours. The average appears to be about eight hours nightly.

The important thing to remember is that, where energy levels are concerned, too much sleep can be as detrimental as too little. If you oversleep on a regular basis, you can bring a new meaning to lethargy. In some cases this habit can even weaken your heart.

Figure out the amount of sleep you need to feel refreshed. Stick to that level as often as possible. If you have to have a late night, make up for it by sleeping longer the next evening. Do not make a habit of getting into sleep debt. You can only make up so much before you throw your body mechanisms into a state of emergency.

SUGAR

Yes, sugar is our number one energy thief. It's true you get an initial burst of pep when you take in simple sugars, but this is short-lived. Far better to take in complex carbohydrates so that the energy is "time-released." That is to say, energy is created slowly over a longer period rather than with a rush (only to be followed by an equally fast drop). Candy, chocolate, soft drinks, and a zillion other sugar-loaded goodies are the enemies of energy. Other than providing calories sugar has no nutritional value, and it promotes tooth decay faster than you can say "Ouch!" in the dental chair.

CAFFEINE

Some bodybuilders enjoy their pre-workout coffee. The caffeine sets us up for an explosive workout. Caffeine (found in coffee, tea, and colas) is a pick-me-up. It can increase alertness, coordination, and concentration; and like carbohydrates it can prevent fade-outs and increase a person's stamina during vigorous exercise. But moderation is the key. Caffeine depen-

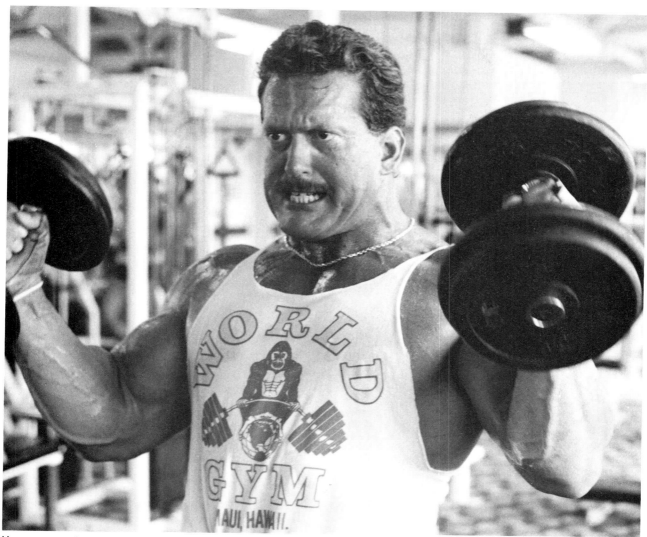
Hammer curls—a World Gym secret for bicep development.

dency can lead to severe anxiety, nervousness, sleeplessness, headaches, and uneven energy levels. Drink no more than four cups of coffee a day and you should avoid the typical overuser's highs and lows.

YOUR WORKOUT ROUTINE

Make sure your workout routine isn't sedentary. So many bodybuilders perform supine bench presses, seated behind-neck presses, incline bench curls, lying triceps, seated thigh extensions, lying leg presses . . . . Every exercise is static. If you want energy, you have to earn it. Make your routine a dynamic flurry of muscle building. By all means perform sitting and lying exercises, but mix in a few multijoint energy-burning movements such as high-rep squats, power cleans, rows, and standing presses.

It's also a good idea to get your body accustomed to change. Switch your workouts now and again. Don't allow yourself to get locked into certain rep patterns year after year. Perform a variety of reps—low, medium, and high. Keep your metabolism guessing and tuned by regular change.

PARTYING

Overpartying can poop you out faster than anything. Chances are that when you party you drink too much, inhale too much smoke (whether first- or second-hand), eat junk food, and stress your body beyond the normal fatigue boundaries. Plan a strategy. Don't stay up till dawn just because you're with friends over a weekend. Promise yourself a decent night's sleep and make sure you get it. Rather than wait for the wee hours when everyone gets hunger pangs and opts for hamburgers and fries, make sure you eat quality food before you start socializing. If you eat just before partying, you will find it easier to resist the party junk. As the social event winds down, hold on until you get home—and then you can get back to quality nutrition again.

AEROBIC EXERCISE

Get moving. The energy-boosting effects of vigorous exercise are well-known to bodybuilders. If you feel your weight training is not contributing much to your overall energy levels, perform some aerobic exercise two or three times a week—anything that keeps your heart pumping above its normal rate for 20 minutes or so. A brisk walk, jogging, bike riding, rowing, stair climbing, swimming, dancing, or your own choice of self-designed aerobic movements. Don't push yourself hard at first. Work into the habit. Pretty soon you'll be known as the kid on the block with energy to burn!

THE PUMP—METABOLISM

Metabolism comes from the Greek word "metabole," which means change. One way to bring about change is through progressive-resistance exercise, which nowadays means weight training and using machines with weight stacks and pulleys. "Constructive change," says Charles Gaines, author of *Pumping Iron*, "is what bodybuilding is all about."

All advanced bodybuilders seek what's known as "the Pump!" Arnold Schwarzenegger liked to say it was better than sex. "A pump gives a feeling better than coming," said the Oak. I always thought this to be a bit of an insult to one's sexual partner, but Arnold made his point, as always. He is not the kind of person who will bore you. His words always have a way of being remembered.

Is a pump necessary for growth? No. Any top bodybuilder could drop down on the floor and perform 50 push-ups and get a humungous pump. But he wouldn't grow from it. Conversely many trainers fail to pump up in the biceps, or shoulders, or back—and still enjoy increased gains in mass.

But a pump (achieved through quality training with substantial to heavy resistance) is a good *indication* that you have "got to the muscle." But let me emphasize that you have to obtain a pump legitimately. That is to say, the muscle should be gorged with blood, feeling tight and big, but it must get that way through hard,

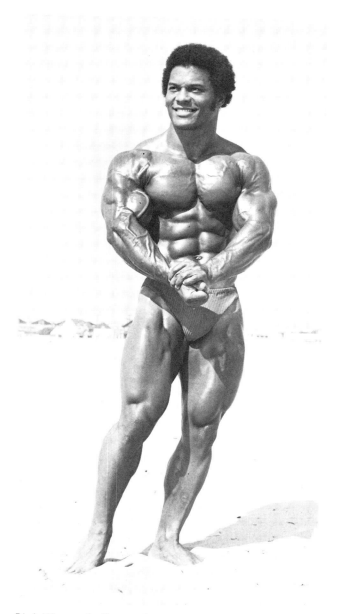

Rick Wayne in the early years.

103

quality sets of meaningful exercise.

If you get to the stage where your muscles never seem to pump up, even though you work them hard, look to your diet, choice of exercises, frequency, and repetition patterns.

DIET

Inadequate food (insufficient and/or of poor quality) will hold back your ability to get a good pump. When your muscles are flushed tight (pumped) it is the result of a lactic acid buildup and blood rushing to the area to feed the muscles being trained. Less than optimum nutrition will put a stranglehold on both your pump and the willingness of your muscles to grow.

EXERCISE CHOICE

Can't pump up? Then change around one of your exercises. Let's assume that you normally perform the following routine for your biceps.

Barbell Curl	5 × 8
Incline Dumbbell Curl	4 × 10
Seated Dumbbell Curl	4 × 10

If you are not managing to pump up with this routine, why not perform another biceps exercise (preacher curls?) instead of the seated dumbbell curl. In fact, it might be a good idea to perform seated dumbbell curls one workout and preacher curls the next. The first two exercises of the routine could stay the same.

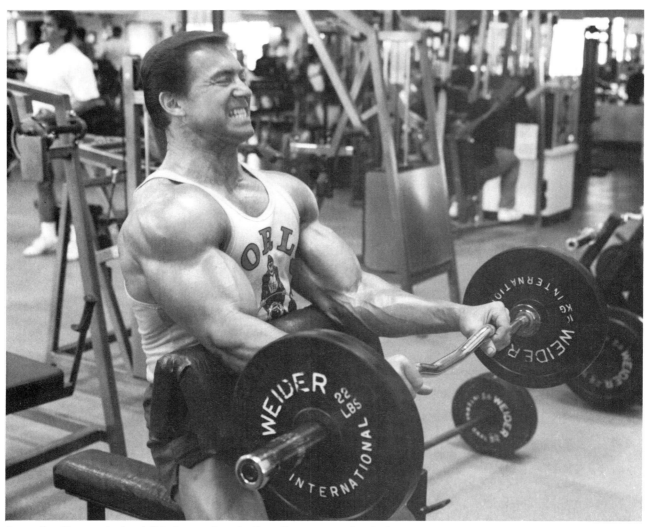

Larry Scott popularized this form of curls, thus the names Scott Curls on the Scott bench.

This rotating of one exercise for each body part can be just the difference you need to maintain regular muscle growth.

FREQUENCY

The more times a week you train a muscle, the less likely it is to pump up. Muscle growth is optimized by training each body part twice weekly. Training three times a week can be beneficial for short periods, but you are courting failure if you train each muscle group three times a week over a long period.

Tom Platz currently squats once a month. He does 50 reps and gets an enormous pump. But he is not trying to add size. He simply wants to maintain mass. On his normal leg days (twice weekly), he performs thigh extensions and leg curls, about eight sets of 15–20 reps. Old-time strongman, Fred Howell, has often stated: "The less you train, the more you gain." In my opinion, there is some truth to this, but let's not go to extremes. What is true is: "The less you train the more you pump." But we have already agreed that a pump isn't vital for growth. It merely acts as a good barometer to indicate when the muscle has finally got the message that you mean business!

REPETITION PATTERNS

We have already agreed that a quick set of 50 floor dips will give even the most hardened pro bodybuilder a great chest pump—yet we unhappily concede that this will not lead to pectoral growth. Nev-

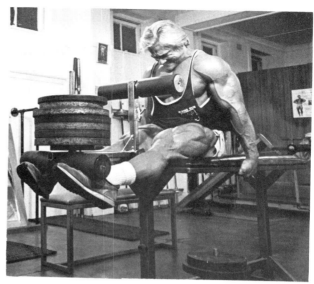

The Golden Eagle during one of his mind-blowing leg extension sets.

ertheless, you should vary your rep patterns to encourage a pump. But before you actively seek to drum up a pump, you must pay your dues with concentrated, quality training. In most cases this translates to four or five sets (sometimes up to eight) per exercise, using 8–12 repetitions, and heavy resistance that really challenges the deepest muscle. If at the end of this hard-core training you still have not achieved a pump, you can lower the resistance considerably and perform 15–25 fast, strict reps to literally force the blood to the area. As you complete this final set the lactic acid buildup may cause you to stomp your feet or gurgle and grunt as the burn takes hold. Try not to scream out. After all, you will be growing, and that's what it's all about. Right?

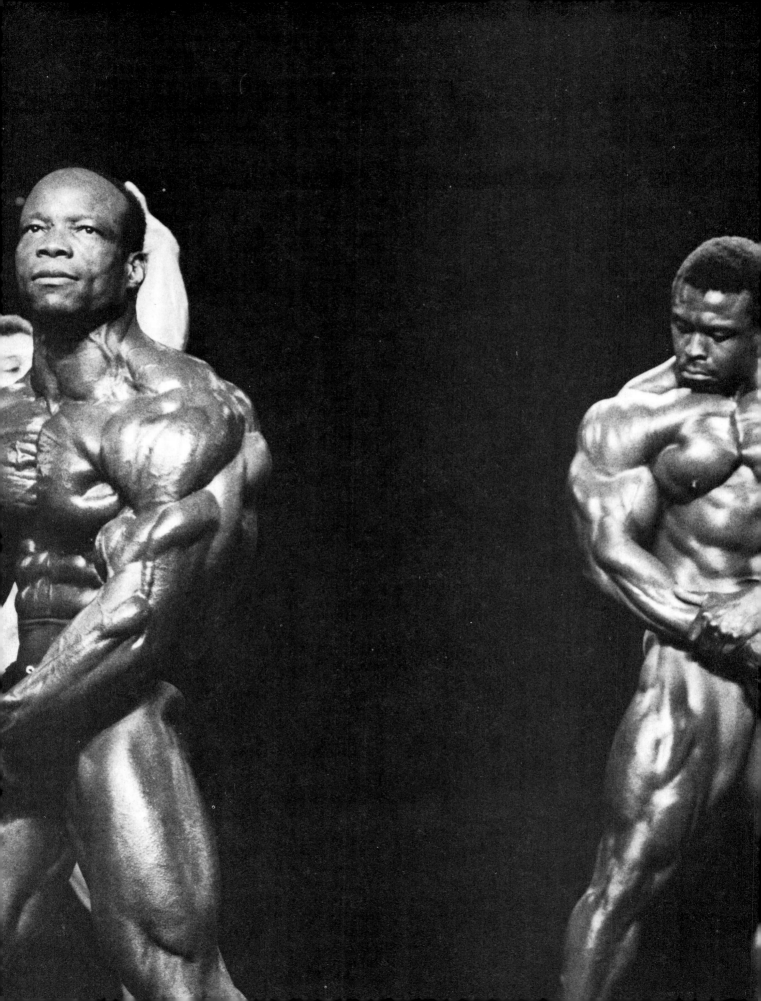

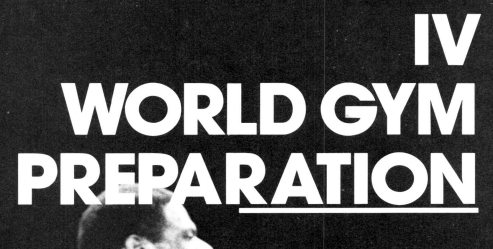

IV
WORLD GYM
PREPARATION

- RIPPING UP
- ENTERING THE SHOW
- POSING

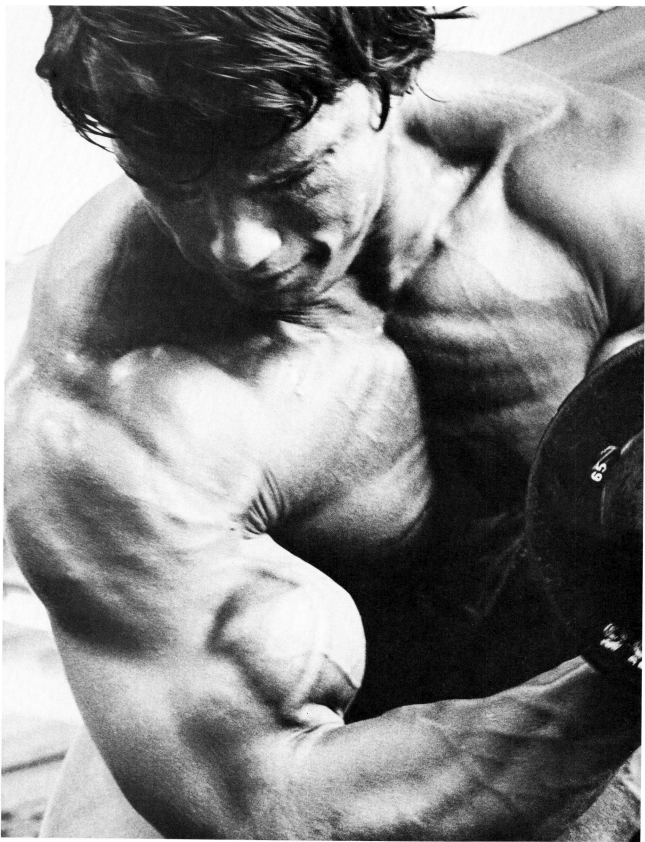

Unbelievable!

RIPPING UP—COMPETITION CUTTING

When preparing for a competition, you really have to set your mind in motion. It's the only way you can succeed. When you know the date of the show you are going to enter, that's the time to program your mind in every aspect of positive training. But don't wait until you start preparing for an upcoming competition before applying a positive mental approach. You should review the mind over matter techniques to help you in all phases of your training, including off-season workouts. Certainly you won't make great gains unless you apply yourself mentally. Tom Platz, following Arnold Schwarzenegger's example, says: "Nothing compares with the mind when it comes to power. If you fail to apply your mental abilities, your fullest training potential will not be realized. In fact, you may not gain at all. Your body always follows the course set in by your mind, so you must program your brain positively to achieve bodybuilding success."

That's what ripping up is all about. And it's not easy. For a long time now I have been aware that just about anyone can train with weights. Almost anyone can get big, but only the dedicated "survival of the fittest" types can follow through with a supertight diet and rip up their bodies to make that quantum leap to real impressiveness at competition time.

Preparation for competition admittedly starts in the gym, but the event is won or lost at the dining room table more than on the gym floor. Many have sought that cut-to-ribbons definition while eating a poorly balanced diet, and as a result they have left themselves bereft of training energy and dangerously unhealthy during the period just before the show date.

It's currently agreed that dieting too harshly (drastically restricting calorie intake) causes loss of muscle mass as well as fat; in some cases you can lose even more muscle mass than fat. Often, under these conditions, metabolism slows down and the body holds on to the fat. This is the body's way of conserving energy; when calories are *drastically* reduced, an alarm switch is thrown, and the metabolism slows down automatically.

It is true that one should be at or slightly below one's ideal competitive weight seven to ten days before the show, rather than trying to diet away body fat the last week. Many make the mistake of starting their diet too late and end up starving themselves during the last week. This seldom works because muscle mass is lost and it invariably leaves loose rolls of skin. Worse, sometimes you are left with loose rolls of fat. This does not occur if training intensity is kept up and a more balanced diet is followed.

Further, bodybuilders have labored under the premise that the more lean and dehydrated the system the better they will look. What they fail to realize is that human muscle contains fat and water, both

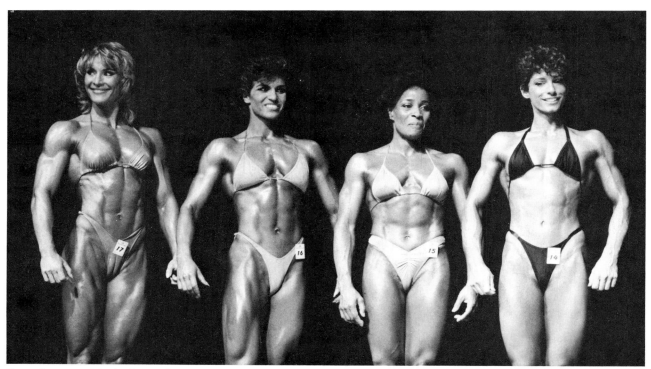

Cory Everson, Marjo Selin, Carla Dunlap, and Penny Price.

of which contribute to muscle rotundity and shape. What an aspiring competitor has to do is get rid of fat and water from under the skin rather than from inside the muscle. Controlling the water in your body is important. It can mean the difference between winning and losing. There are two main ways in which water can be pushed into muscle cells to give maximum size and hardness.

1. Altering the electrolyte balance across the membrane of the cell so that water will pass from extracellular areas to intracellular areas.
2. Precontest carbing up, thereby forcing the muscles to absorb large amounts of glycogen along with three times as much water.

The water content of a cell is regulated by the relationship of the amount of potassium inside the cell to the concentration of sodium outside the cell. When there is an excess of potassium, water is sucked into the cell, where you want it. When there is an excess of sodium, water is drawn out of the cell and deposited under the skin, where you most definitely don't want it.

By clever manipulation of the potassium-sodium balance, a bodybuilder can encourage more water to deposit itself inside the cell. Quite simply this can be done by drastically reducing sodium intake while increasing potassium consumption in the form of concentrated supplements. This works well for about three days, and then the body discovers the trick and rights the wrong. Nature has a way of bringing these things back to the status quo.

Twelve days before the event, eat reasonably high levels of sodium (take salt with your meals). This will encourage your body to hold on to more potassium (to keep nature's sodium-potassium balance) than it might otherwise do. When you finally reduce your sodium levels (during the last three days), you'll have naturally high levels of potassium, making the potassium-sodium imbalance more pronounced and drawing more water into muscle cells. Caution: sodium loading doesn't mean you should consume large amounts of salt, nor does it need to be

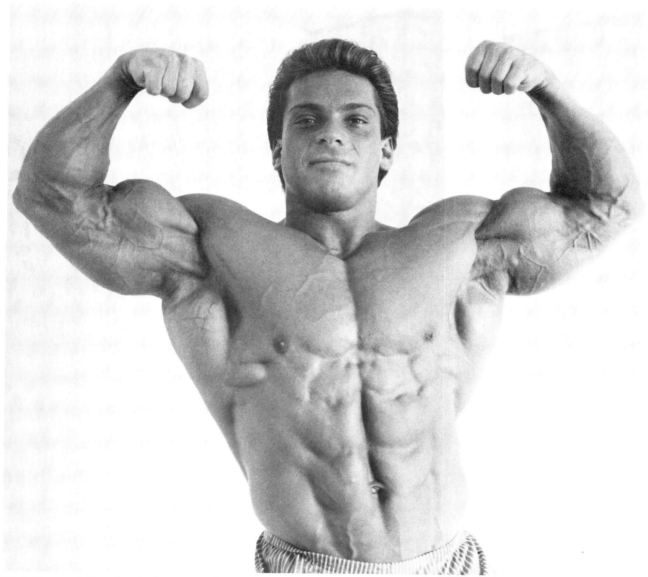

Rich Gaspari, the day before a contest.

done for long periods of time. Too much salt on a regular basis can lead to high blood pressure and heart problems. Sodium loading is merely a short-term trick of the trade to help you rip up with maximum size.

While reducing all sodium intake during the last three days before your competition appearance you should simultaneously take potassium supplements. No one can tell you exactly how much to take, but the rule of thumb is that a 200-pound bodybuilder should take about 100 milligrams five times a day (daily total of 500 milligrams). Take potassium with food; it

should never be taken on an empty stomach.

Hard training builds both muscle and capillaries to give you size, but additional size can be obtained if you can persuade your muscles to store more glycogen. Hard training, especially in conjunction with a severe diet, tends to deplete the muscles of glycogen. They look flat. Because the body is programmed to overcompensate when there is a depletion, it will be predisposed to storing extra amounts of the glycogen you ingest. With careful dietary manipulation you can make this overcompensation even more pronounced, first by restricting

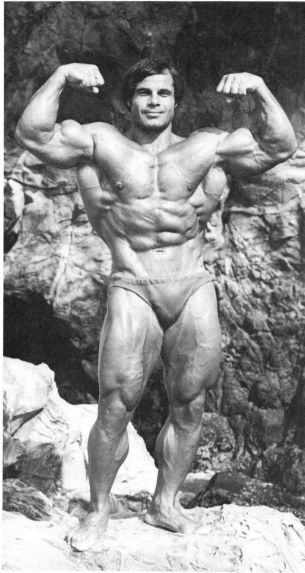

Franco is as hard as the rocks he stands on.

bankrupt foods, during this carbing up period. Check the sodium content of everything. If you are not positive about the sodium content of a food or drink, don't swallow it! Drink distilled water these last three days. You don't have to limit your water intake, because at this time you are trying to draw it into the muscles. The high carb intake will cause you to soak up plenty of water, because you've created a one-way street in which water is being

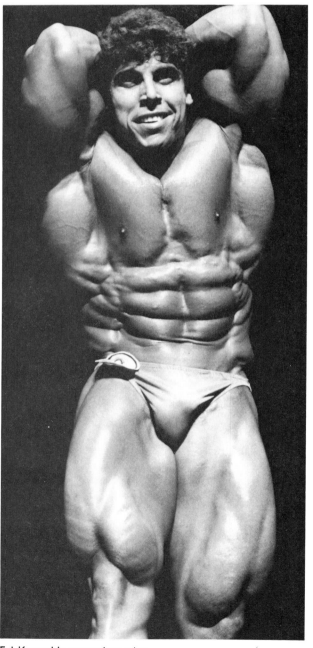

Ed Kawak's amazing abs.

your carbohydrate intake for a period of three to four days, right down to zero if necessary, and then during the last three to four days before showtime ingesting small amounts of carbohydrates (potatoes, rice, or yams) every few hours during waking hours. The body requires at least 70 hours, sometimes longer, to fully carb up. Don't begin the process later than the Wednesday night before a Saturday show. Never carb up with simple carbohydrates like sugar or ice cream. This could cause your body to secrete large amounts of insulin, which in turn can retain water under the skin. Avoid junk, nutritionally squeezed into the muscle cells and cannot leak out and deposit itself under the skin. Excess water is merely eliminated in the urine.

How much training should you do during the final few days? Different bodybuilders have different methods, but the consensus is not to train at all on Thursday, Friday, or Saturday (show day) until the time you pump up before going on stage. But make a point of posing three times a day on the Thursday and Friday before the show.

Should you eat other foods when carbing up? Yes, small amounts of protein and some fresh green vegetables and an occasional apple or banana. Keep your fat consumption to a minimum. Don't take saunas or diuretics, but if you are decidedly bloated during the last days of preparation, merely limit your liquid intake and do some light aeorbics such as stationary bike riding or fast walking.

COMPETITION COUNTDOWN SCHEDULE
SUNDAY TO WEDNESDAY EVENING
(FINAL WEEK)

- Regular high intensity, medium- to high-rep workouts.
- Low-key aerobic activity.
- Moderately high sodium (salt) intake.
- Low to zero carbohydrate intake.

WEDNESDAY NIGHT TO SHOW TIME
(SATURDAY)

- Three daily half-hour sessions of intense posing.
- Light aerobics (if needed).
- Little or no weight training.
- Regular carb-up periods (one potato each 1½ hours).
- Low to zero sodium intake.
- Plenty of distilled water at intervals.
- Potassium supplements with food.

ENTERING THE SHOW

We all are being judged all the time, but can there be anything so nerve-wracking as being judged in pose briefs?

With today's clothing styles anyone with a little imagination can pass muster with his or her contemporaries. But being judged at a physique contest is definitely somethin' else!

The answer to anything involving the unknown is *preparation*. Having made up your mind to enter a competition (or at least allowing someone to talk you into it), you now have to do everything in your power to make the best showing possible. Bear in mind that whether the judges admit it or not you are being judged on your whole appearance. That includes not only your body but your face, your skin, your posture, your tan—even the way you walk and the fit of your costume . . . everything. It is your duty then not only to build your body the World Gym way but also to double-check your preparation list so that you are secure in the knowledge that, win or lose, you have done your best.

TANNING

Don't leave getting a natural tan to the last minute. Even Florida, California, or the Mediterranean can dish out days of continuous cloudy skies. Use either natural sun or a sun bed to acquire your color, and start at least six weeks before the competition. But even dark-skinned peo-

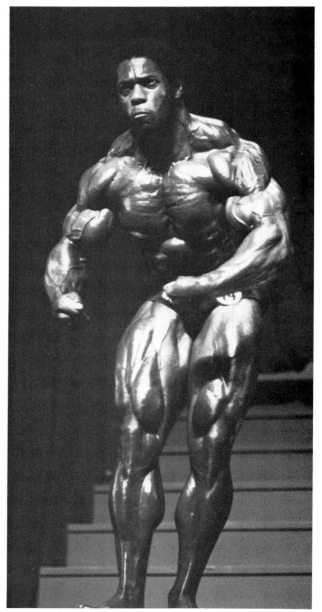

The world's best most muscular a la Bertil Fox.

114

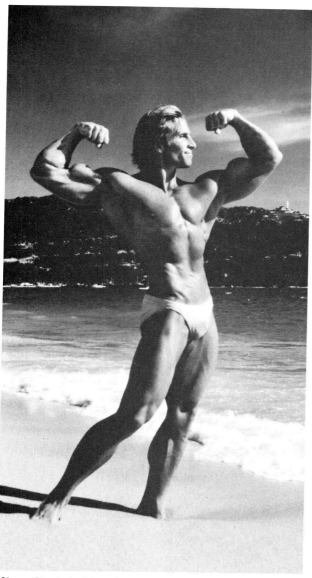

Steve Davis in his prime.

YOUR COSTUME

Make sure your costume complements both your physique and body color. Women and men should make sure that the genital area is completely covered. Women should practice posing with the costumes they will be wearing at the show. Otherwise you could be in for a shock. Your double biceps pose may cause the costume to ride up and expose your breasts. This has happened numerous times and can cause embarrassment you can do without.

OIL

Before going on stage apply oil to your entire body, taking care not to spill any on your costume. The best oil is almond (available at health-food stores) because it has a skin-tightening effect that will help your appearance. Too much oil, especially on a smooth-white-toned physique, can give a mirror effect, reflecting back to the judges and giving a poor overall image. However, if you are really evenly (and richly) tanned, and especially if you are ripped to the bone, use plenty of oil. A little too much is definitely preferred to too little. A well-oiled body will give you the edge over your competition.

HAIR STYLE

Many women wear a different hairstyle for the prejudging than they do at the evening show. At prejudging the hair is often drawn back or set in a ponytail to give a fit, athletic appearance (making the shoulders look wider, too).

Evening-show hairdos for women are often more styled. In fact, several of the top pro women have their own hair dressers accompany them to shows.

Hairstyles for male bodybuilders are usually pretty businesslike. Curiously, even at the height of the long-hair fashion in the seventies, few long-haired bodybuilders fared well in international competition. Even bearded bodybuilders have (for

ple like Juliette Bergman, Marjo Selin, Danny Padilla, Ali Malla, or Rachel McLish need more than a sun-bed tan. The added ingredient is Dy-o-Derm, a brush-on liquid that will give you a deep, dark color. This product is available through mail order ads in *Flex, Muscle and Fitness*, and *MuscleMag International.* (Cory Everson is one supplier, at 7324 Reseda Blvd., Suite 208, Reseda, Ca., 91335.) Warning: if you are serious about looking your best, you will need several eight-ounce bottles of Dy-o-Derm, because you will have to paint on several layers during the days leading up to the show.

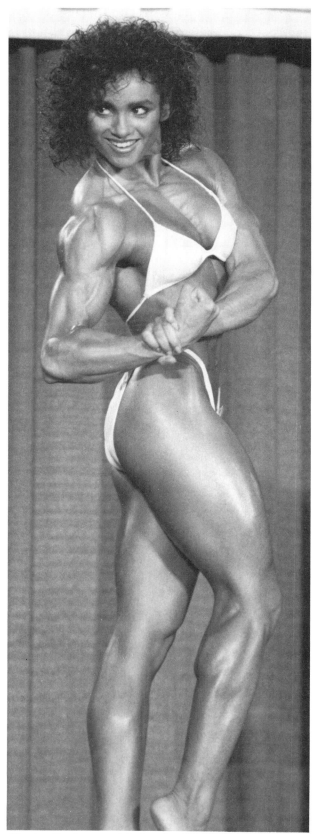

Gladys Portugues lets her hair down for the evening show.

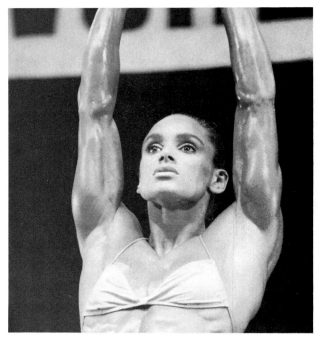

Gorgeous Gladys has her hair up for the prejudging round.

whatever reason) failed to dominate the really big shows. The lesson is simple. Don't allow your hairstyle to detract from your physique. Whatever styles happen to be in vogue, one cannot argue with the fact that "shortish" or "combed-back" hairstyles accentuate a bodybuilder's shoulder width, overall body size, and athletic appearance. Men should also remove all body hair. Use shaving soap and a standard blade razor. If you are very hairy, you'll need plenty of fresh blades to do the job without searing the skin.

INITIAL IMPACT

If you are in shape for a show, your job is to make sure the judges notice you from the second you walk on stage. Too often ripped-to-shreds competitors are overlooked in the early rounds because the judges are busy comparing "name" bodybuilders. When the judges finally notice that the person in question is in fantastic shape it's frequently too late for the person to pull up in points enough to place at the top. If you are in shape, *show* the judges that you mean business. When called out for comparisons, *get* noticed

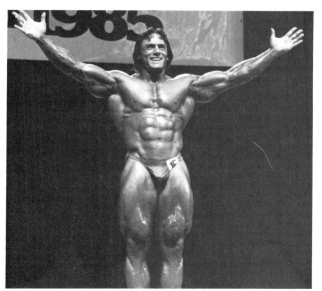

Muscular development is wasted if it can't be properly shown on-stage—Bob Birdsong at the completion of a great Olympia routine.

quick. Hit the poses the second they are called and telegraph your enthusiasm—blatantly!

BE PREPARED

Take everything you'll possibly need to the show. Two towels, two costumes, oil, touch-up makeup, a small mirror, a sweat suit, slippers, warm-up coil cables (strands), distilled water. . . .

Above all, don't wait until the last week before a show, to buy oil, tanning creams, or costumes. Things being what they are, something will go wrong, and you'll be in a state of panic during those last all important days when all you really should be concerned with is reaching an all-time physical peak.

POSING—THE ART OF SELF-PROJECTION

Bodybuilding encompasses so much more than just lifting weights to add muscle mass. Today one has to be a show-biz expert as well, not to mention the arduous diets needed to rip up for a show. Yes sir, posing is an art, and if you want to win you just can't afford not to practice your routine endlessly.

Posing starts in the bathroom mirror, but ideally you should have two or three full-length mirrors set up in such a way that you can study your posing from all angles. If you just pose your upper body while brushing your teeth before hopping into bed, you won't develop much of a routine. Chances are you'll never learn how to pose your legs properly.

In most events today the judging is done *before* the actual show, either during the afternoon preceding the evening performance, or the day before. The format is pretty much the same in every country. Competitors are asked to line up on stage and are then compared with one another in groups of two, three, or four. You may all be asked to stand sideways, face the same direction, frontward or backward. Then you will be compared to others in different "compulsory" poses. Frequently these are the front double biceps, the side chest, the front thighs and abdominals, the back lat spread, and the back double biceps.

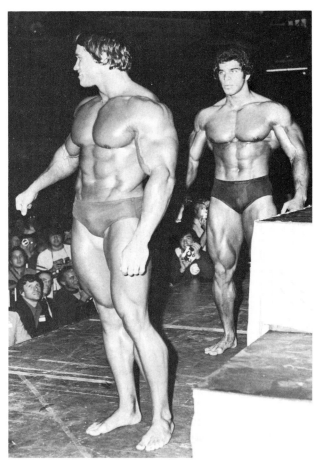

Arnold and Lou in competition.

Judges seeking to rank competitors in order of merit will compare them in identical poses. This can take considerable time and be very nerve-racking, not to mention physically demanding. To add to the anxiety, competitors not being called

118

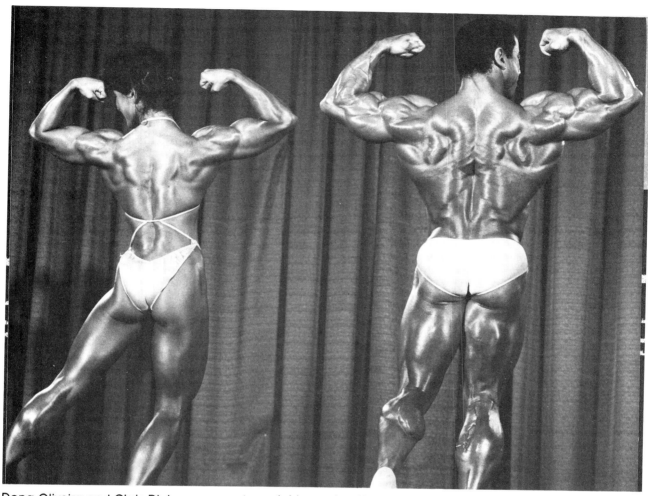

Dona Oliveira and Chris Dickerson pose in matching colors that complement their skin colors.

out for comparisons, but who are standing on stage, should "keep tight" because the roving eyes of the judges are ever-vigilant—and if they catch you with a lazy posture, thighs and abdominals not tensed when the person next to you is as tight as Scrooge, you may lose points.

The next round is usually the *free-posing* section. This is your opportunity to show your individuality, usually to your own choice of music. When free-posing you do not *have* to perform any prearranged poses; in fact, you can avoid poses that don't suit you and cover up weak points by omitting certain stances. Let's assume you have a poor V-shape from the

back. You have to give away this secret in the compulsory section, but there's no reason to shove your weakness down the judges' throats a second time.

Don't know how to free-pose? Imitate the pictures in the magazines for starters, and then make a habit of attending local shows. Next on the agenda is to buy videotapes of the various Olympia competitions. Play them over and over. Learn how each champ projects the body beautiful—and pose along with them.

If you have access to a video camera, set it up on a tripod, stick your favorite music on the record player, and pose your heart out. Chances are you'll feel better than you

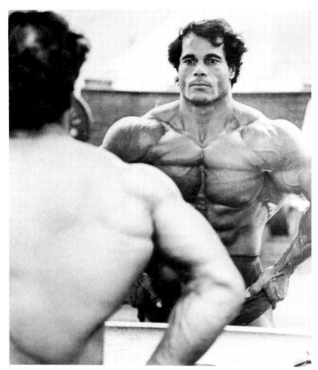

The artist scrutinizing his work.

look. But everyone has to start somewhere. In time you may become the expert, and others will play your tape to learn posing secrets from you.

Always try to improve your posing. Make changes with a view to perfecting the entire routine. Try changing the pace, simplifying your transitions between poses. Practice smiling, or at least not grimacing. If you are short and stocky, it may not be a good idea to copy poses more suited to tall champions. The same works in reverse. Tall competitors can seldom perform poses more suited to shorter bodybuilders.

Remember that all is not lost if a particular pose doesn't look good when you first do it. Keep practicing the pose, either in the gym after your workout or at home. You may grow into it. At one time Frank Zane couldn't perform an effective lat spread, yet eventually, with constant practice, it became one of his most impressive poses. He never gave up. With practice, Lee Haney turned a *weak* side-chest pose into a work of art. And Mike Christian turned an ordinary most-muscular into the most

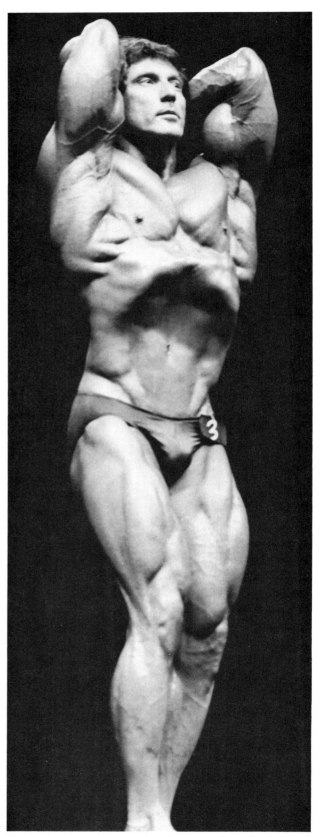

Frank Zane was known for stage routines that would bring down the house.

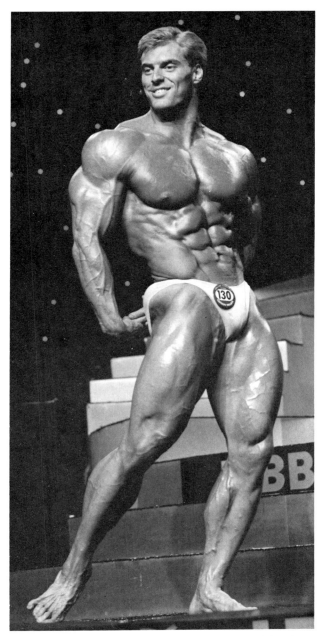

Berry DeMey has made his muscular good looks pay off for him in a successful modeling career.

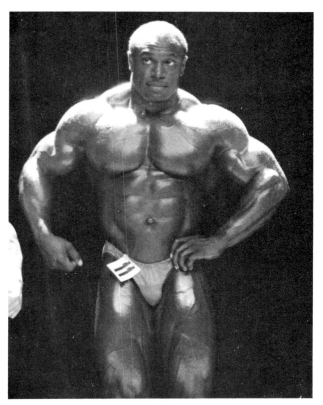

Lee Haney waiting to be crowned Mr. Olympia for the third consecutive time.

awesome stance in modern bodybuilding . . . with practice.

If you're lucky enough to get into the top six in a competition, you'll find yourself in what is termed as the posedown.

The head judge will line up the six finalists on stage, making sure there is adquate room to perform lat spreads, etc., without hitting or bumping the person next to you. You are then given two minutes to pose. This is the time when you show your most muscular poses. Forget those artsy, beautiful poses. They will neither be noticed nor appreciated, because in a posedown the finalists invariably end up bunched together trying to upstage one another, and there is no room for artistic poses. *Beef wins out in a posedown.* If you move forward to the edge of the stage during a posedown, be sure there is enough light to show your muscles to advantage. So often, finalists rush to the front of the stage only to fade out because there is little light there.

During a posedown, try to hold eye contact with the judges. Avoid full back poses because eye contact is lost, and a back pose cannot hold up when compared to a front pose. If everyone does back poses together, that's another matter. But it never works out that way in a posedown.

Never walk away from a posedown. Invariably the winner is left at center stage, still posing when the judges call a halt. Those who walk off early are forgotten and fail to place well.

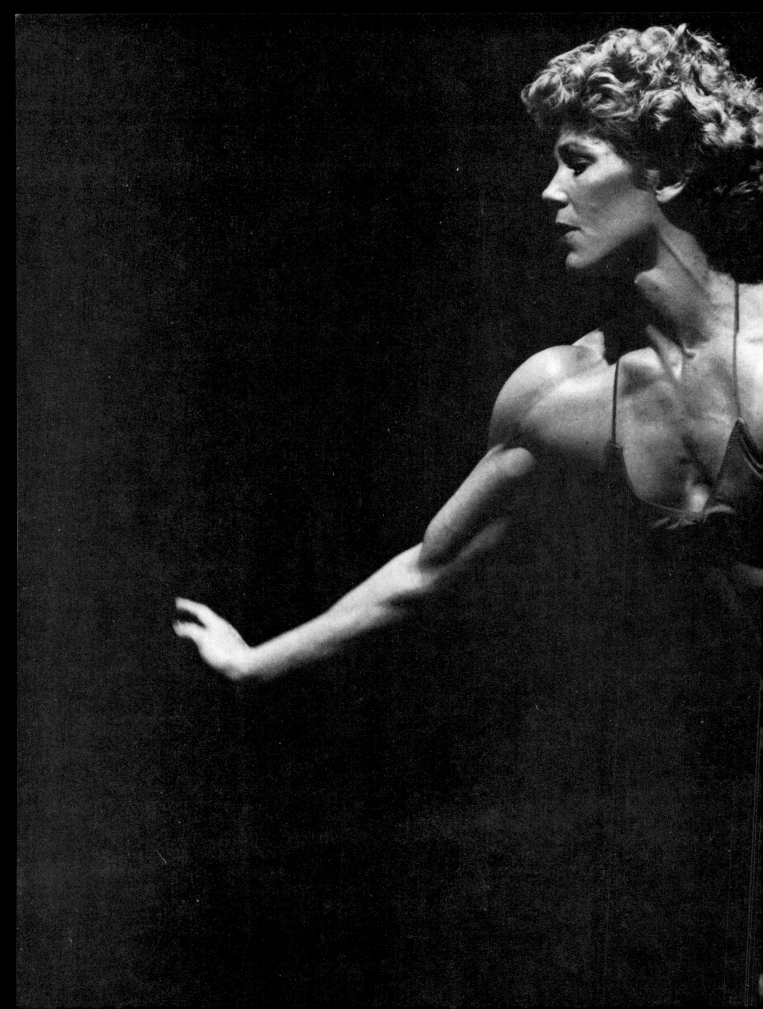

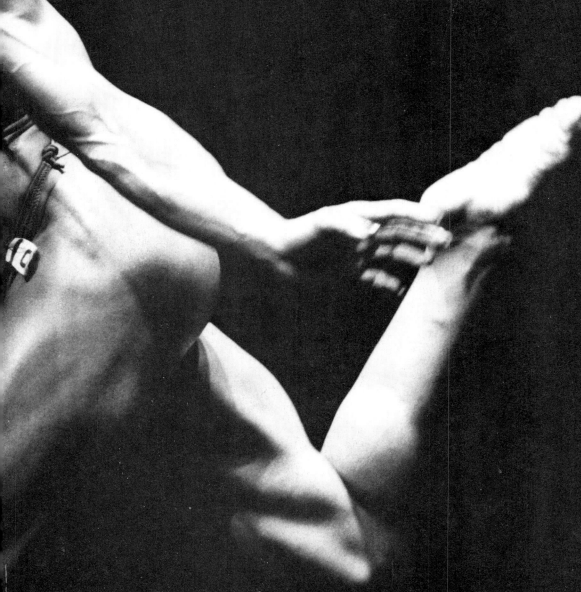

V
WORLD GYM
PERSONALITY

- THE P FACTOR
- MUSCLES MAKETH MONEY

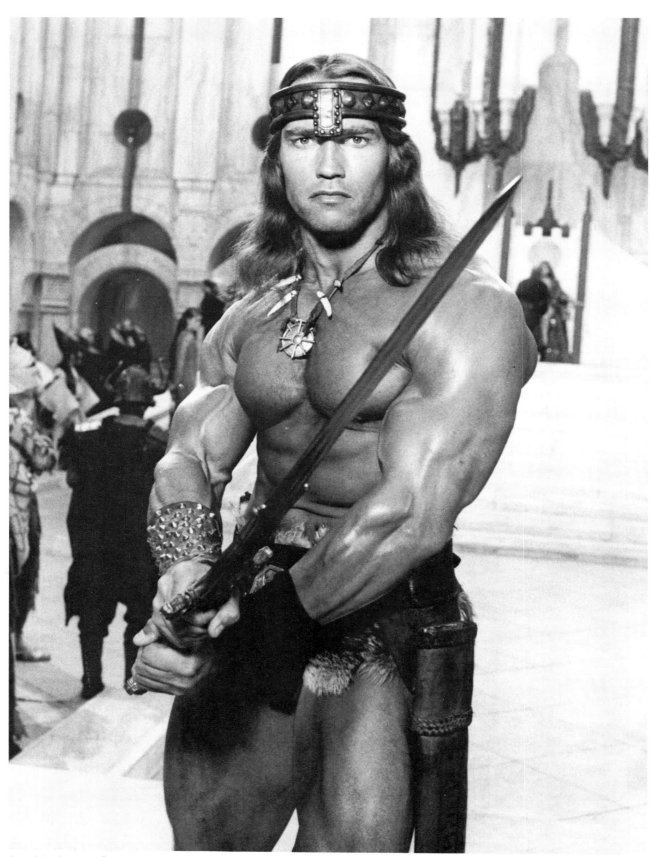

Arnold playing Conan at the beginning of his film career.

THE P FACTOR—PUBLICITY BRINGS FAME

Publicity is a factor that no serious competitive bodybuilder can afford to ignore.

The late Andy Warhol has been misquoted ad infinitum as having said, "Everyone will be famous for at least one minute." In fact, he said, "Everyone *should* be famous for at least one minute." Acquiring fame is a difficult proposition at best, and rarely drops into the laps of the unsuspecting.

Fame boosts your earning power as a competitive bodybuilder, your ability to attract work, and to a degree your ability to win competitions. To a degree in the latter category because you still have to come across with the goods—but fame can give you that winning edge. Fame means having people know your name, your face, and your physique. And the only way to achieve fame is through publicity. The P factor.

Publicity should be part of any bodybuilder's arsenal. Just as important as posing trunks, tanning pills, and aminos, publicity can give you that quantum push to success. Lack of it can kill your career.

The value of publicity should be no secret. The sport's top names have utilized publicity from the start, building up names and reputations that capture the public's attention and imagination. *Arnold*, *Franco*, *Platz*, *Gaspari*, *Rachel*, *Gladys*, and *Cory* are all names synonymous with success. They all have turned their careers into big-money endeavors.

All have been in the public eye through magazines, guest posing, and even movies. Arnold Schwarzenegger hired a publicity agent at the start of his career. He was always ready with quick one-liners on the talk shows and was always asked back. He became a celebrity because people remembered his personality, not just his physique. Tom Platz became a publicity machine, grabbing press coverage whenever he could, emphasizing his "nice guy" image. Hardly an issue of a bodybuilding magazine hits the newsstands without some coverage of Rich Gaspari. Rachel McLish utilized her sex appeal through articles and posters to bring a new image to women's bodybuilding. Brian Moss, President of Better Bodies Management, pushed Gladys Portugues through all the avenues, mainstream as well as physique magazines, legitimizing the female bodybuilder in the public's eye. Cory Everson works with the best photographers and writers to ensure her image is that of the consummate professional. Other famous bodybuilders were created solely by publicity, never having entered, let alone won, a contest. The *Barbarians* and *Teagan Clive* come to mind in that category. I myself never won a Mr. America or Mr. Universe title, but my name is synonymous with the gym business. . . . I hope you're starting to get the idea.

THE P FACTOR—AMATEURS

As mentioned earlier, publicity will not win a contest. You still have to train, diet,

125

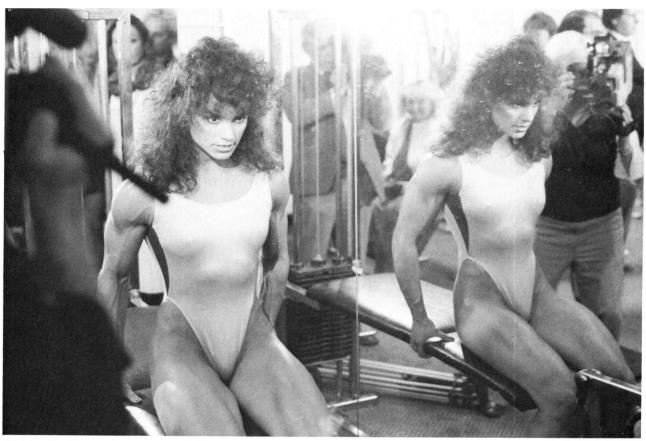

Gladys Portugues has successfully brought muscular femininity to the masses by appearing on several non-bodybuilding magazine covers.

tan, pose, and all the other prerequisites of competition. Publicity *will* give you an edge. The judges will be looking for *you*. Publicity makes you a personality rather than a faceless physique. The rest is up to you.

As a rookie you are caught in a "catch-22" situation. Want to win a competition? Get some publicity. Want some publicity? Win a competition. What to do?

You must approach your publicity campaign like a business. Some investment, both in time and money, may be required in order to garner a pay off. First, you want photographs taken. With no offense to Uncle Henry and his Instamatic, you want good-quality photographs. Unless you have friends in the photographic trade, contact a professional photographer. Tell him what you want and ask his price. Many photographers will be willing to shoot your portfolio for a small fee plus

some photographs for their files. Shop around.

You'll need posed shots outdoors, studio posed shots, training shots, and some standard model material. The last requirement is up to you and the photographer's imagination. Browse through the various magazines and see what's in vogue. Remember, the more varied the activities, the more people relate to your personality. And that's what makes photo editors take notice. Make sure you're in shape, tanned, and well groomed for the sessions, and that's about it, other than a recommendation that you shoot color transparencies and black-and-white negative film. Most magazines and editors require color slides and 8 × 10 black-and-white glossies. The best photographers in the business are Steve Douglas, Mike Neveux, John Balik, Harry Langdon, John Running, Paul Goode, and World Gym's own Art Zeller.

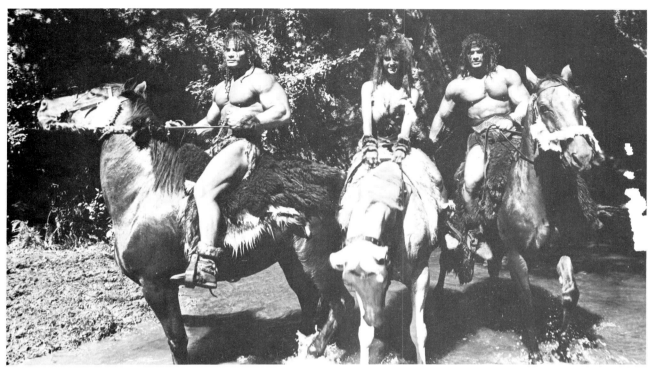

The Barbarians during a scene from their new movie.

Next, contact a writer. It's always best to use a pro from the start. You want to impress editors with your professionalism. Again, check out the magazines and see the route most *good* writers are taking. Have the writer interview you with these articles in mind. Make sure you cover a lot of turf in your article. Lots of information and a fresh angle will grab an editor's attention faster than the old sets-and-reps route. Try to tie in the article to the photographs to make an interesting package.

Having done all that, send the lot to the various magazines (you can find the address at the bottom of the masthead. Also check the magazine's policy on unsolicited material). An important point to remember is that nothing ticks off a publisher more than to see duplicate articles and photos in a rival magazine. Take the time to edit the photographs and articles so that each publisher gets a totally different package. Make sure every parcel contains a polite cover letter, a self-addressed, stamped envelope, your article, your 8 × 10 glossies, and your slides in vinyl sleeves—don't expect a photo editor to go through those little yellow boxes. That's the fastest way to end up in the reject pile. There is no guarantee that your story will be published, but an impressive photo story certainly stands a chance.

Another route is to contact the magazines directly, inquiring when staff writers and photographers will be in your town. Larger than regional competitions

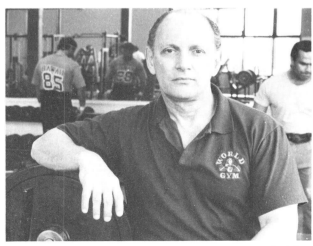

Master Photographer Art Zeller—one of the World Gym gang.

usually attract a contingent from the various magazines, if in fact your town hosts such an event. Inform them of your current status and your availability for shoots and/or interviews. Send the editor a quality physique shot of yourself to whet his appetite.

One method to grab the attention of art directors and editors is to have a head sheet printed up. This is a page with a photo or photos, along with your name, vital stats, and where you can be contacted. These can be mailed to magazines, agencies, and related manufacturers, informing them of your availability for modeling, endorsements, or just about anything of this nature. You can also contact local manufacturers in person. Put together a professional-quality portfolio for this, one that consists of the best photographs you can have done. Update your portfolio periodically, and be extremely harsh in *your* critiques. They will. Also,

have a resume printed up that you can leave after these interviews. Try to develop working relationships with the various trade people. Get to know them, first by learning their names in the media and then contacting them by mail or in person. Several amateur bodybuilders I know are bringing in a few extra bucks while cultivating these important connections.

Above all, be polite and personable to everyone you meet in the industry. A well-placed friend can further your career markedly. A well-placed enemy can damage it irreparably.

THE P FACTOR—PROFESSIONALS

You're a pro, you've won your fair share of titles, and the magazines, promoters, and manufacturers are approaching you for your services. You've made it and can afford to act with the aloofness of a true celebrity. Right? You couldn't be more

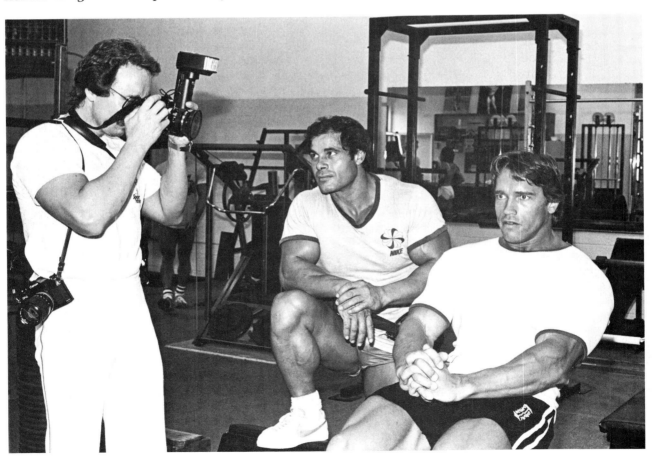

Arnold and Franco are always the focus of attention.

wrong. Your bodybuilding career is in a constant state of flux. New faces consistently spring into the limelight. Old faces frequently disappear from the public's view. You've got to fight to keep your face, physique, and reputation at the front of the pack. Publicity can develop and keep a legion of staunch fans and admirers—a fact that any show promoter can't afford to overlook when he's deciding on a guest poser for his show. Publicity makes your name bankable; it assures box office success. Your endorsement is worth a few more zeros on that paycheck. Lack of publicity can cause you to fade into obscurity, in fame *and* earning power.

Physique stars come and go at a blistering rate. The people who can keep the public's attention stay. Tom Platz is a master of publicity. He freely admits that it's his bread and butter. His fame keeps the jobs and cash coming in. It's made him one of the wealthiest bodybuilders on the planet. Tom always shows up for a photo session. Seldom turns down an interview. His squeaky-clean image, created by Tom and promulgated by the magazines, has captured the public's imagination. And Tom maintains his publicity machine to keep it that way.

None of this should be a secret. Amazingly, it is. I am amazed by the number of bodybuilders who do not show up for photo sessions and interviews the day after a competition because they were teed off at their placing. Being in fantastic

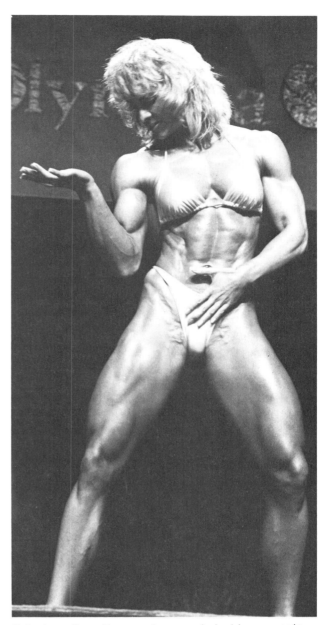

Fabulous Cory Everson has marketed her muscle extremely well while continuing to win the Ms. Olympia.

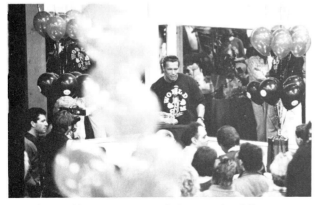

Arnold making a ceremonial speech at the opening of the new World Gym in Venice, California.

shape, these people could, with a few hours of work, guarantee a year or more's worth of publicity. But they don't show up. It's a one-hand-washes-the-other affair with the magazines. Your physique helps sell the mags, the mags help sell your physique. Simple as that.

Many pro bodybuilders are overlooked by the media, and consequently by the public, because they are simply not aggressive enough in their publicity cam-

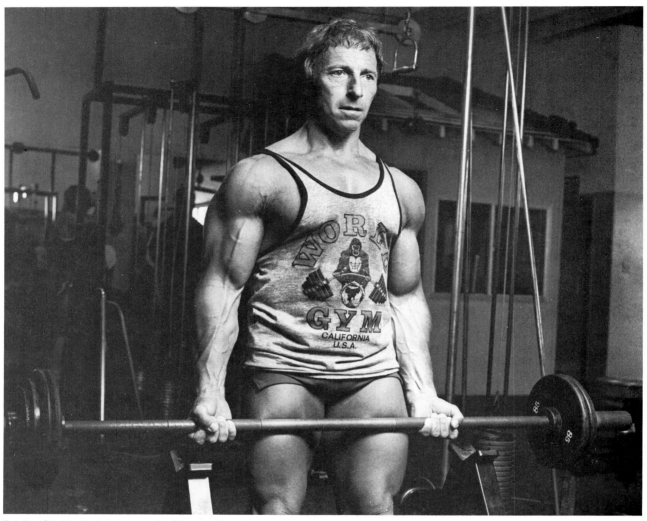

Eddie Giuliani during a set of barbell curls.

paigns. Pros also must take the time to arrange interviews, photo sessions, and interviews with the media. The industry people are sometimes too busy to look you up. You must chase *them*. Remember, a little bit of PR work goes a long way. If you can't spare the time and energy to do the footwork, hire an agent or manager. Brian Moss was one of the main reasons behind Gladys Portugues's rise to stardom. He was never off the phone, arranging sessions, interviews, and doing other PR work for Gladys. He also handled all the contractual negotiations. One thing to keep in mind is that a manager or agent will take a cut of your earnings. Usually between 15 and 20 percent. Do not sign a long-term agreement with an agent. A year

or two at the most. You may not be happy with the way you are represented.

Publicity can also give an edge to the pro bodybuilder in his competitive career. In the top pro ranks the difference between the top placers is miniscule. The physiques are so similar that the smallest factor can sway the judges. Just as a darker tan, smoother posing, or a more confident manner can influence the judges, so can publicity. The judges read the magazines and trades—they know who the top names are. With a successful campaign blitz, they will be looking for you, your name etched in their minds. Many impressive bodybuilders have been overlooked in the first round. True, the judges will eventually notice the good phy-

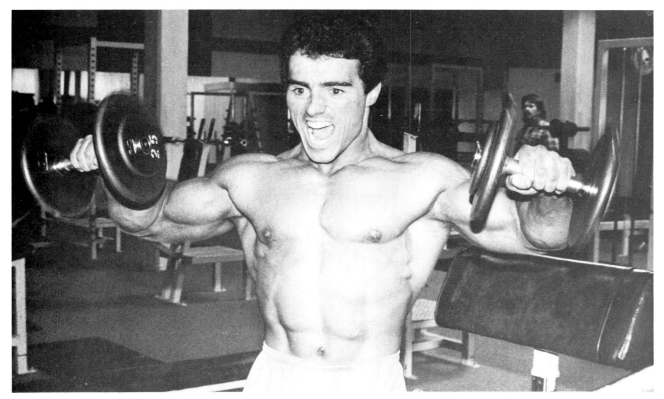

Lat raises are essential for fully developed delts.

sique of an underpublicized competitor, but by the second round it may be too late. Again, publicity can't win a show for you alone, but it can certainly help. As a pro you must approach your training, diet, and publicity as a business. Develop a relationship with the various people in the industry. They can only help you.

You may also need a professional head sheet and resumé to assist you as you try to break into the mainstream areas of advertising and media. Contact the photographers you have worked with. More than likely they will be glad to lend or give you some photographs. These head sheets can be mailed to agencies, casting offices, and manufacturers along with your resumé.

Whether you are a pro or amateur bodybuilder, developing a publicity campaign comes down to two factors: time and work. That is your investment. Your pay-off is the fame that is associated with publicity, and the financial gain. By now, you should know that publicity is like dirt; throw enough of it, and some will stick. It worked for Andy Warhol.

MUSCLES MAKETH MONEY—CASHING IN

We all love bodybuilding for its own sake. In fact, the last thing on many hard-core purists' minds is the thought of making money. But as we get older the importance of having to support ourselves becomes a reality. And if we get married and start a family, the financial aspect becomes even more crucial. We *have* to make a living. We then have two choices: we either make a living doing regular work, such as office, manual, creative, or selling, or else we make a living from the sport we love. There are arguments for and against making a living from your hobby. The negative argument is that by turning your bodybuilding into your life's work you may lose the joy in training. Many a time Joe Weider has told me that he is frequently too busy to train. This always brings a smile to my face because Joe has millions of dollars, and if anybody in the world can "afford" to train, he is one who can.

Despite running World Gym and its many franchises around the world, I still find time to train, and I always have. It's just a matter of setting time aside for the job. Personally I'm a believer in making a living from a hobby — and I've tried both ways. Much of my life was spent as a merchant seaman. Somehow when you turn your hobby into your life's work you consolidate both. You make more money because you understand the business;

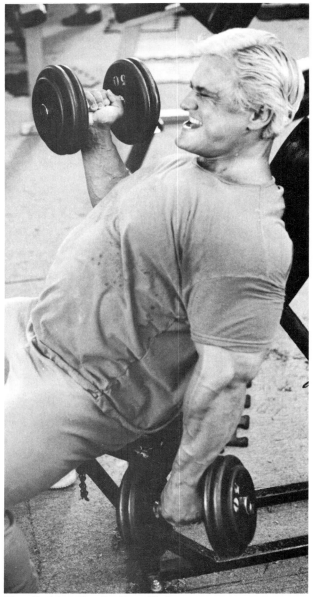

The Golden Eagle, Tom Platz.

132

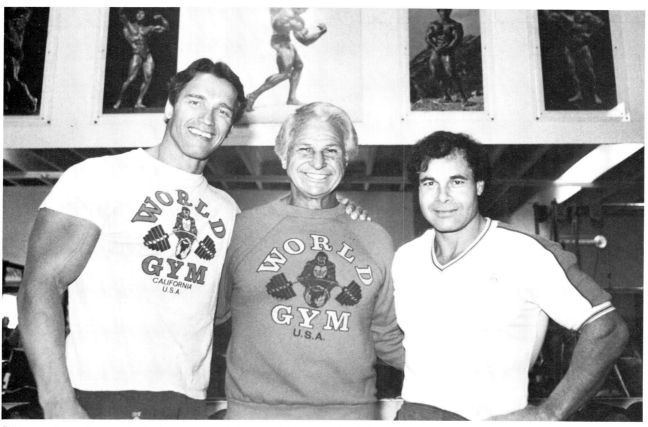

The very backbone of World Gym and the World Gym principles.

and you benefit in your training because your business knowledge has spilled over to give you more insight into training. One hand washes the other.

ONE-ON-ONE TRAINING

This is probably the most common way to make money from bodybuilding. One-on-one is merely putting someone through a workout; it involves designing the program, working out a correct nutrition plan, and actually standing by while the client performs each set. Many clients want more than someone to put them through a workout. They want someone to talk to, to share their problems with that are totally unrelated to bodybuilding. Sometimes this can be a drag, especially when you're psyched-up for a serious workout.

Double Mr. Olympia Franco Columbu charges a set fee to shape up top film stars for certain film parts. His fee sometimes runs into tens of thousands of dollars for a three-month training program. Unlike most one-on-one training experts, Franco says that the best way to train someone is to train with him, set for set. "It helps pace the workout," Franco says with a smile. Obviously a trainer with several daily clients can't physically go through a workout each time one of them trains. One film star that Franco has trained successfully for his roles is Sylvester Stallone. If you compare Stallone's physique in *Rambo* or *Rocky IV* with that in *Rocky*, you'll see what I mean.

What do regular one-on-one trainers charge? The fee is usually between $15 and $100 a workout. The average is $35 a workout. You don't have to be a champion to be a one-on-one trainer. Most agreements are arranged personally through flyers or small posters placed on the gym's bulletin board: "One-on-one trainer available for men or women. $35 per hour. Call: 555-1234." Some people located in big

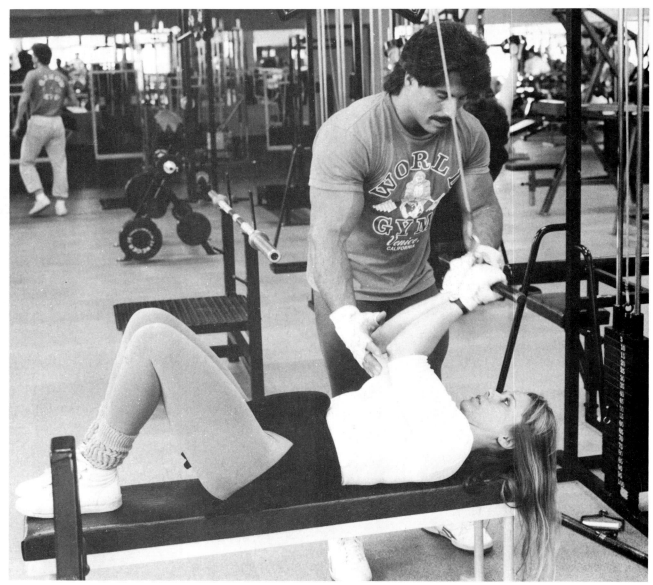

Many muscle athletes use their expertise in one-on-one training sessions at a gym for extra money.

cities such as New York, Chicago, Toronto, or Los Angeles place classified ads in bodybuilding magazines and get good response. Many make a good living with just three or four regular clients a week.

MODELING

Pursuing a career in modeling while bodybuilding can be lucrative. Certainly Gladys Portugues succeeded, as have Marjo Selin, Rachel McLish, Erika Mes, Reggie Bennett, Ray Valente, Eric Hunter, Tommy Terwilliger, Ming Chew, Jon-Jon Park, and Bob Paris.

The steps to modelling success are:

1. Build a symmetrical, well-proportioned, eye-catching physique.
2. Become proficient at how to behave in front of a camera in different situations. A modeling course may be necessary.
3. Get publicity through the various bodybuilding, fitness, and health magazines. Send in articles and photos.
4. Acquire an agent who understands both the modeling and

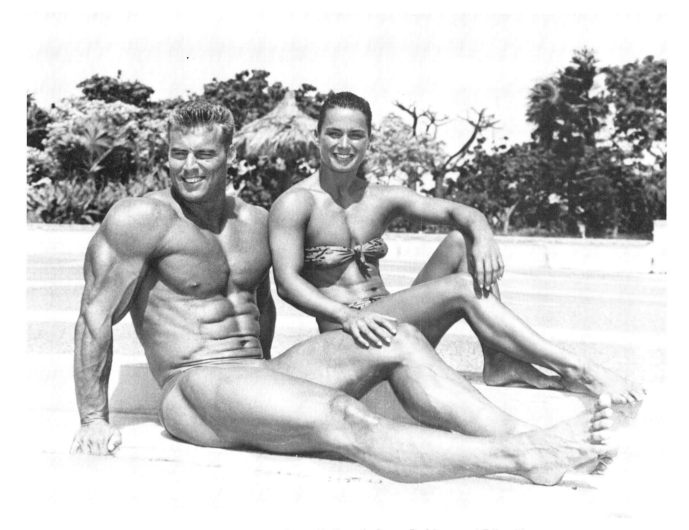

Both make money modeling and guest posing—Holland's Berry DeMey and Erika Mes.

bodybuilding businesses. Brian Moss of Better Bodies in New York comes to mind.

5. Be on time for appointments, so that those who use you know you are a reliable professional.

Mail Order

The beauty of mail order is that you can work from your own home. You can fill orders from your kitchen table if you like. Many fortunes have been made with bodybuilding mail-order products. The great successes include Vince Gironda, because he was one of the first name bodybuilders to offer good instruction through his training manuals; Larry Scott, who was the first Mr. Olympia to produce body-part booklets; Arnold Schwarzenegger, who built up his name by winning everything in sight; Rachel McLish, who was the first top woman to offer hot women's items; Mike Mentzer, who captured the bodybuilder's imagination with his dynamic writings on "Heavy Duty" principles; Tom Platz, who has steadfastly worked to promote himself in a professional manner, and who rightfully has been termed the world's most dedicated trainer; Cory Everson, who is an undisputed world champion; and of course the King of Bodybuilding Mail Order . . . Joe Weider. All of these people have grossed hundreds of thousands with muscles-by-mail offers. Not a few have grossed millions.

There are some rules in mail order:

1. Only sell those items that cannot be bought easily in stores.
2. Select items that are not too costly to mail — T-shirts, books, courses, clothing, pose wear, supplements, videos, etc.
3. Have a professional graphics house design your ad. Make sure the ad has a picture of your product and contains plenty of selling copy, with a catchy headline. Use an order coupon, and if possible include a phone number where credit card orders can be phoned in.
4. Always fill your orders promptly and

make sure that all complaints are answered. When a customer returns a product for whatever reason, make sure a full refund is sent immediately.

COMMERCIALS

Fit, energetic, well-built men and women are always in demand for TV commercials. Some companies want superbuilt pro bodybuilders, others want lighter-built athletes to portray fitness and zest. Among those bodybuilders who have hit pay dirt with TV commercials are Frank Zane (Miller Beer), Franco Columbu (Vitalis), Rachel McLish (Bally Health Clubs), Arnold Schwarzenegger (7-Up), Ming

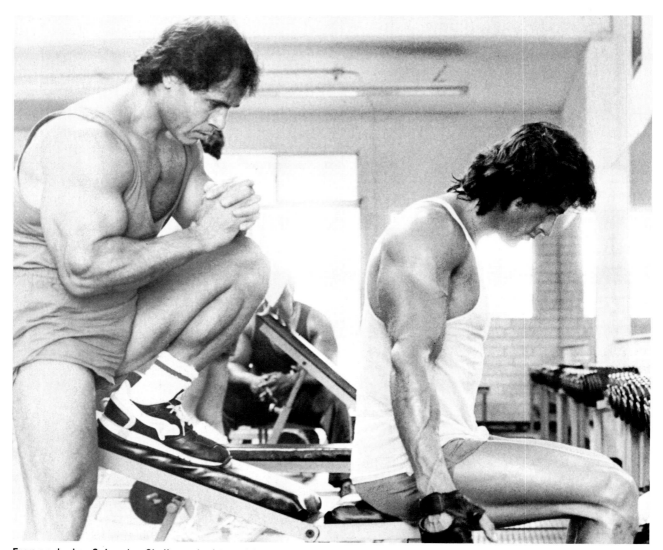

Franco trains Sylvester Stallone to keep him in Rambo shape.

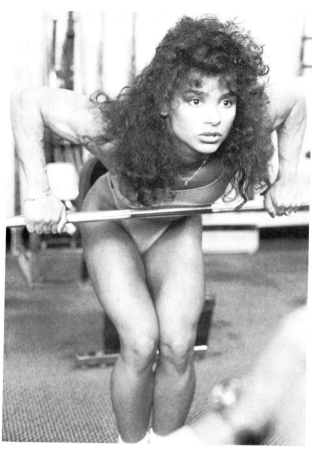

Although no longer competing, Gladys still bodybuilds to maintain the form that is in such great demand.

Chew (Diet Coke), Tim Belknap (Kodak), Lori Bowen (Miller Lite), Gladys Portugues (Nike), and Mohamed Makkawy (Super Fitness Spas). Making it in commercials usually requires more than just a body. Some degree of fame from winning competitions or appearing in bodybuilding mags is usually needed. You should also try to get plenty of experience in front of a camera. Directors hate working with bodybuilders, or anyone for that matter, who can't perform simple actions on direction, such as laughing, smiling, grimacing, standing confidently, walking and running smoothly, etc.

OPENING A GYM

Most bodybuilders dream of one day running a gym. Surprisingly, not many pro bodybuilders run their own gyms. Lynn

Conkwright does, as do Roy Callender, Bob Jodkiewicz, Jusup Wilcosz, and Sergio Oliva. Those who used to run their own gyms but sold out to take life easier include: Bill Pearl, Reg Park, Arnold Schwarzenegger, Rachel McLish, Steve Davis, and Tony Emmott.

The gym business is not as easy it may seem. It's not just a matter of renting a big area, putting in some weights and apparatus, and waiting for customers. Most gyms fail because they are underfinanced. There's not enough money to go around— to pay the rent, to cover wages, to take care of advertising, to pay for top-notch equipment.

A conveniently located gym, with well-designed, hard-core apparatus and free weights, set in an airy atmosphere offering ceiling height, natural daylight, and clean surroundings, can do well. But gym hours are long, and keeping everything humming can be hard work. Various gym franchises are offered, one of which, of course, is World Gym. There is ample proof that starting a franchise with a well-known name is the safest and the most profitable way to go. There is far less chance of going bust and far more chance of making top money. For those interested in the World Gym franchise system write: Mike Uretz, 1134 W. Olympic Blvd., Suite 275, Los Angeles, CA, 90064, U.S.A.

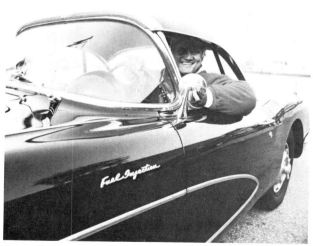

Tom Platz enjoys the fruits of success.

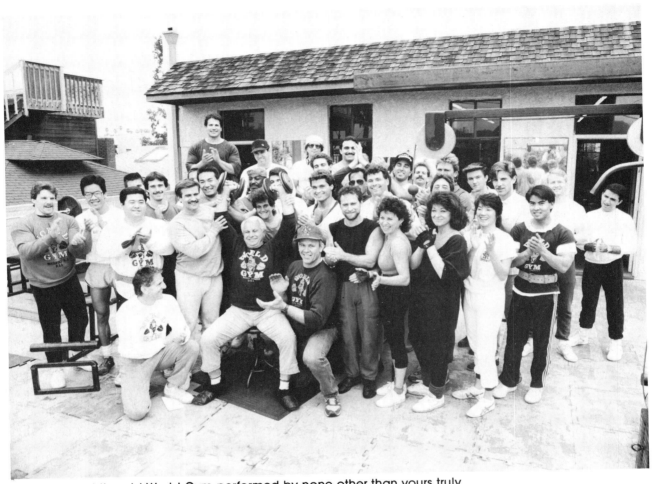

The last rep at the old World Gym performed by none other than yours truly.

ENTERING COMPETITIONS

Today more prize money is being offered to professional bodybuilders than ever before. But it's still not at a level that can give more than a handful a good living. Ironically, some of the greatest bodybuilders in the world don't enter competitions offering prize money they could easily win. During his Olympia wins, for example, Lee Haney could have entered and won every men's Grand Prix (and Mixed Pairs) title going. It would have given him at least another $50,000 to $100,000 a year in direct prize money and spin-off benefits. The same goes for Cory Everson. All she would have to do is walk across the stage at the Skyline Hotel in Toronto, where the Women's World Championships and Mixed Pairs events are traditionally held—and they would hand her first prize.

That's why I admired Arnold Schwarzenegger in his competitive days. He entered every darn competition he could, and even went so far as to invite other pros to enter so that the events would be more exciting.

If you are a young bodybuilder hoping to make a fortune from winning professional competitions, I'm afraid you'll be disillusioned. The prize money helps, but it may not come often enough to keep you solvent.

BOOKS

There are now a zillion books on the market—some good, some bad. Few realize that only a few authors—such as Bill Reynolds, Franco Columbu, Arnold Schwarzenegger, Rachel McLish, and Robert Kennedy—actually make good money. If you are planning to write a book, you

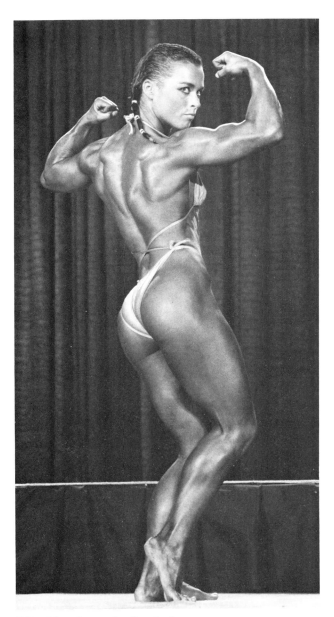

Erika Mes flexes for the judges.

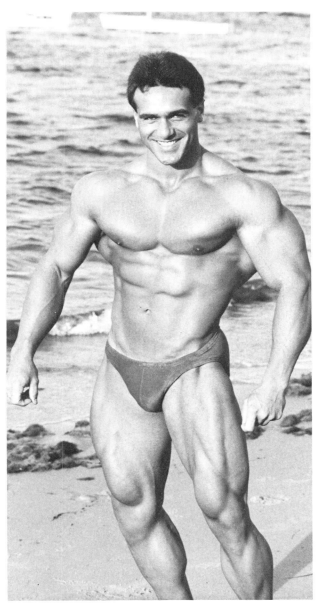

John Terrilli showing fine form on the beaches of southern Cal.

had better be sure that what you have to say is genuinely helpful to the body-builder. Does it really help readers get bigger, stronger, more cut? Are the photos by the world's top bodybuilding photographers? If not, how can the book interest the public? People look for the best, and they will only buy a book if it is the best one on the rack. The usual procedure for having a book published is to contact a publishing house and explain your idea in a brief letter. If they think you have salable material, they may publish your work and agree to pay you a royalty of five to eight percent of all copies sold. A $10 book typically brings an author 50 to 60 cents a copy, which is paid six to eight months after the sale is made.

ENDORSEMENTS

Bodybuilding products sell best when they are endorsed or recommended by other well-built bodybuilders. The bigger

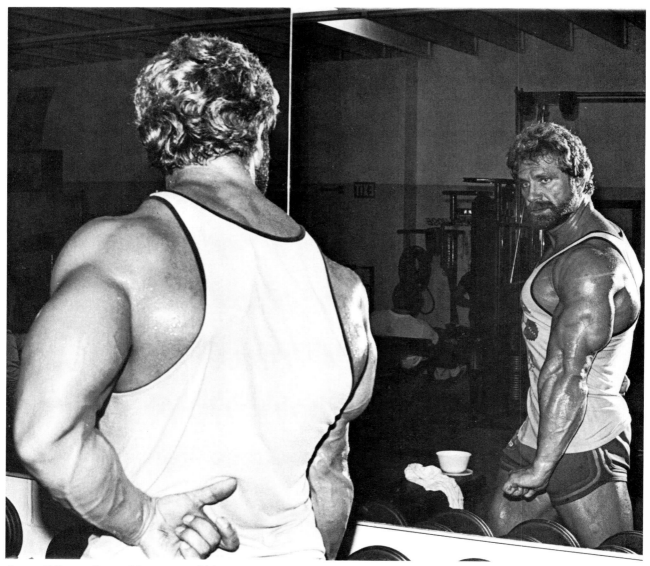

Jusup Wilcosz flexes his pumped tricep.

the name the better the product will sell—and the more a promoter may pay for that name bodybuilder.

Obviously you will not find yourself in terrific demand for product endorsements unless you have won some competitions and been publicized in the magazines, but if you are well-built and on your way to winning, you can be sure that there will be some demand for you in the product-endorsement field.

If you already are a well-built body-builder on the way to the top, there is nothing wrong with contacting a manu-facturer of a product that you like. If you like Nike shoes, write to the company and

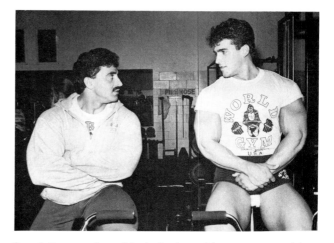

Samir Bannout and Bob Paris get in some aerobics at World.

offer your services. If you've grown on Joe Weider's Megapaks, send him a picture and let him know that you would like to be paid for endorsing the product.

Making money in bodybuilding is largely a matter of taking the bull by the horns and making those initial moves on your own. At first, even though you may have won some important titles, few people will beat a path to your door to hand you money and opportunity. You have to go for it yourself!

QUESTIONS
AND ANSWERS

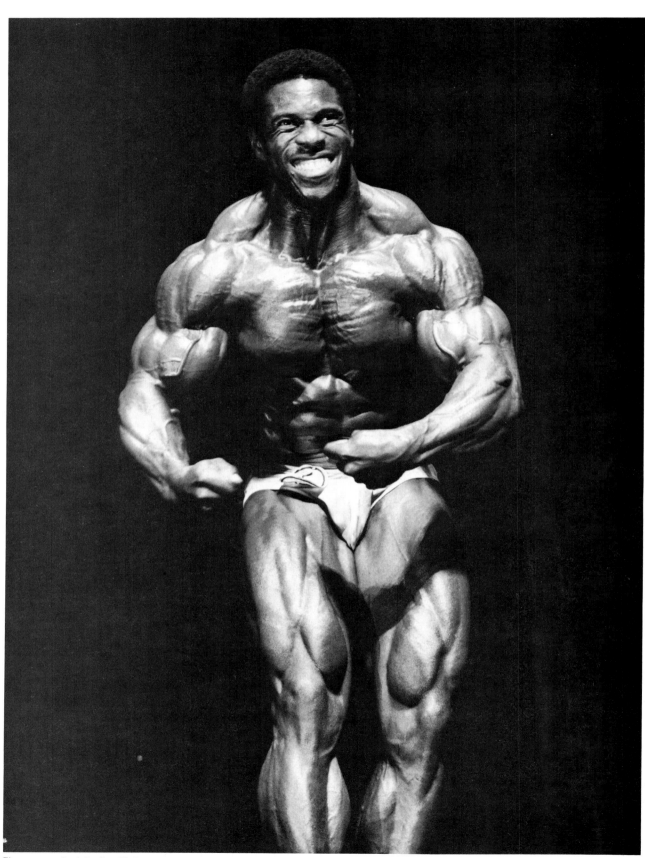

The remarkable Bertil Fox.

BERTIL FOX

Q I once came to your gym and took three workouts over a four-day period. Each time I arrived Bertil Fox had just finished up his training. I never did get to see him train. Can you give me a rundown on how this huge Britisher works out?

A Bertil Fox is like a bulldog in the gym. He prefers exercises such as back squats, bent-over rows, barbell curls, bench presses, incline dumbbell presses, behind-neck presses, lateral raises, standing calf raises—all the basics. Bertil likes to use very heavy weights, and his style is usually pretty loose because he finds that he gets best results from this form of training. I might add that when Bertil trains, quite a few mouths open in admiration and astonishment.

SETS & REPS

Q As long as I have been bodybuilding, I am still not sure about how many sets and reps to do for best results. Please help me on this matter.

A There is no ideal or *perfect* combination of sets and reps. You have to believe this. Obviously, true beginners who've never exercised should only do one set. They should quickly advance to three sets. Intermediate and advanced trainers usually train with the same number of sets per exercise—usually four to six sets for each movement. Large body parts,

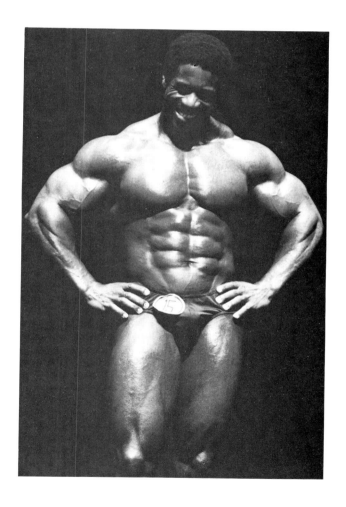

such as the chest, thighs, and back, are often worked with 15 to 20 sets for each area. Shoulders, because they have three distinct areas, are also worked with 15 to 20 sets.

Smaller areas, such as the biceps, forearms, abdominals, triceps, and lower legs,

145

are usually taken care of with 9 to 12 sets.

As for repetitions, this is a matter of personal experimentation. Some muscle areas, such as abdominals, forearms, calves, and sometimes quads, are trained with high reps (15–25), whereas other groups are exercised with moderate reps (8–12). There are exceptions, of course, Franco Columbu, Bertil Fox, and Dennis Tinerino often prefer low reps (five or six per set), while Diana Dennis and Kevin Lawrence, for example, are said to average 30–50 reps on almost every exercise! It just goes to show—one man's meat is another's poison. I should add that some of the World Gym bodybuilders get good results from mixing up their reps. They perform some sets of five or six reps and others of twelve to fifteen reps.

MORE OR LESS

Q In talking to bodybuilders I find two distinct differences in attitude toward making gains. One school of thought insists that muscle-building gains are made from increasing poundage in all exercises. Other authorities tell me that the amount of weight used has no bearing on the muscle's appearance, and is consequently irrelevant. Can you put me straight on this puzzling inconsistency of training philosophy?

A Keeping score of the amount of weight you use in each exercise, and trying to increase the poundage when possible, is a good way to track your progress. Adding more weight gives you a target and a feeling of accomplishment. Beware, however, of allowing your training style to suffer just to satisfy your yearning for more poundage.

It is when a bodybuilder is into the advanced stages of training that poundage becomes unimportant. The bodybuilder is now so familar with his or her body that muscle can be built, shaped, or reduced at will. One trains by *style*, not poundage. Weights become the tool used to create the perfect physique. The champion bodybuilder can use moderate

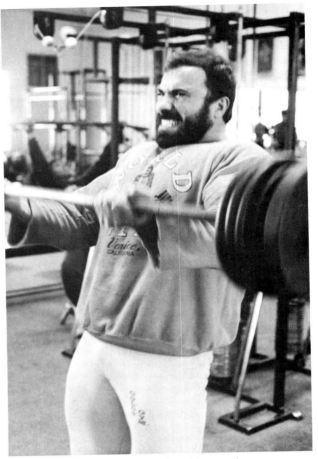

Serious weight for serious development.

weights to achieve results, whereas a less experienced trainer, lacking the knack and sensitivity to his or her biofeedback, can only rely on increasing poundage to log progress.

DUMBBELLS

Q Is there any advantage to using dumbbells over barbells, or vice versa?

A Obviously barbells are superior in exercises such as squats. Two-handed dumbbell exercises are possibly superior to two-handed barbell exercises because they offer, in most cases, a greater range of movement and they force each arm to work independently. However, I am still in favor of using barbell exercises as well. Single-arm dumbbell movements have a definite advantage in that when working one arm at a time you can position your body to maximize stress on that one side, whether you are working your shoulders, triceps, biceps, or lats. In addition, since you don't have to divide your neural impulse (the driving force) between the two sides of your body, you can obtain greater stimulations and contraction, and consequently more growth. This can be demonstrated by the standing barbell press. You may be able to press a 150-pound barbell overhead, and so reasonably calculate that you could press only a 75-pound dumbbell with one arm. However, in all likelihood, you would be able to press 85 pounds or more. The mechanics of the lift change to suit the single-arm movement, plus there is increased nerve impulse. The two together add up to extra stimulation for the area being exercised.

I NEED LATS!

Q I'm having trouble getting my lats to grow. I seem to be at a sticking point. I've tried high reps, low reps, even supersets, but nothing seems to work. How can I get my lats to start growing again?

A I suggest that you take a week off all lat work to rest the area. Then when you start to train your lats again use different types of exercises to hit the muscle fibers from new angles and in different ways—for example, try a chin or pulldown movement, a rowing movement, or a pullover movement. Try three to four sets each of wide-grip chins, bent rows, and bent-arm pullovers, or behind-the-neck chins, T-bar rows, and dumbbell pullovers. Concentrate on isolating and spreading the

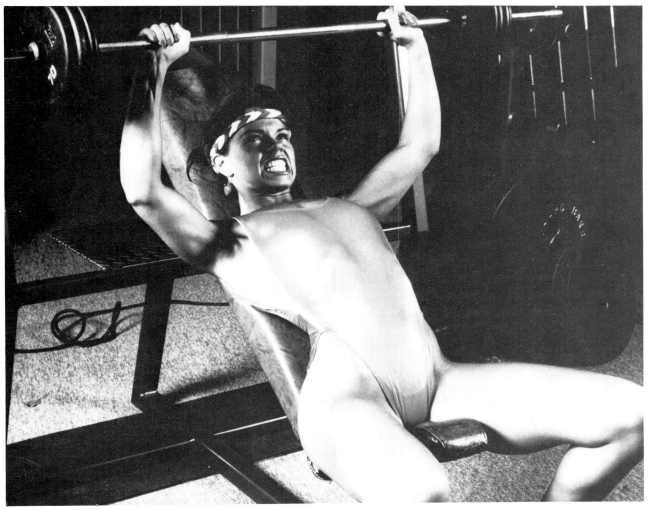

Negrita Jayde, of Canada, performs incline barbell press.

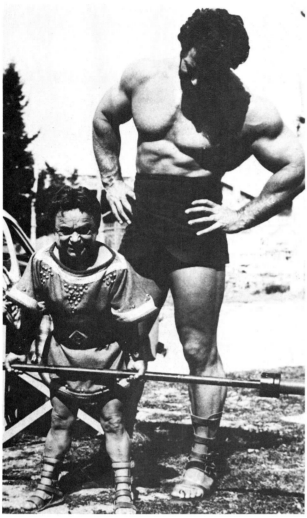

Famous muscleman Reg Park on the set of Hercules with a pint-size admirer.

lats as much as possible with each rep. Also do some lat stretching—hang from a chinning bar for 30 to 60 seconds or grab hold of something and pull back with your body, really giving the lats a good stretch.

GRIP BUILDER

Q I am a bodybuilder, but I also enjoy doing some powerlifting. I am having trouble maintaining my grip on heavy deadlifts. What exercises should I do to build up my grip?

A Heavy forearm work—wrist curls, reverse curls, reverse wrist curls—will help, as will hand-gripper exercises, if you can find heavy-duty ones that provide

enough resistance. Also try heavy weights and low reps on the grip machine. One-hand deadlifts are good, done straddle style, with the barbell between your legs. Also try heavy partial deadlifts on the power rack, holding a heavy weight for certain lengths of time. Set the pins so that you have to lift the bar only a few inches to get it off the pins. You might also want to try pinch-grip exercises. Grab a smooth 50-pound plate with no lip on it and just see how long you can hold it. Also grab a heavy pair of dumbbells and walk around the gym with them and see how long you can hold them. All of the above should give you a grip like any oyster.

TRAINING MISTAKES

Q What do you think is the most common training mistake that body-builders make?

A Without a doubt, overtraining and trying to do too much. Most body-builders don't realize that most of the routines they read about in the bodybuilding magazines are precompetition routines, designed to tear down, not to build up. It takes maturity and intelligence to learn restraint. It's better to undertrain slightly than to overtrain slightly. Always keep something in reserve. In the off-season, I'd recommend no more than six to twelve sets per body part. When training for size, train big, eat big, and think BIG! When training for cuts, train faster, eat smaller, and think CUTS!

TOO YOUNG?

Q Is 13 too young to start bodybuilding? How old should you be to start?

A Thirteen years of age is not too young to start bodybuilding, as long as it is done sensibly. By sensibly I mean not trying to handle too heavy weights that might cause injuries. Actually there is a benefit to starting young. The tendons, ligaments, and bones are still soft, and the skeletal structure still growing, so the

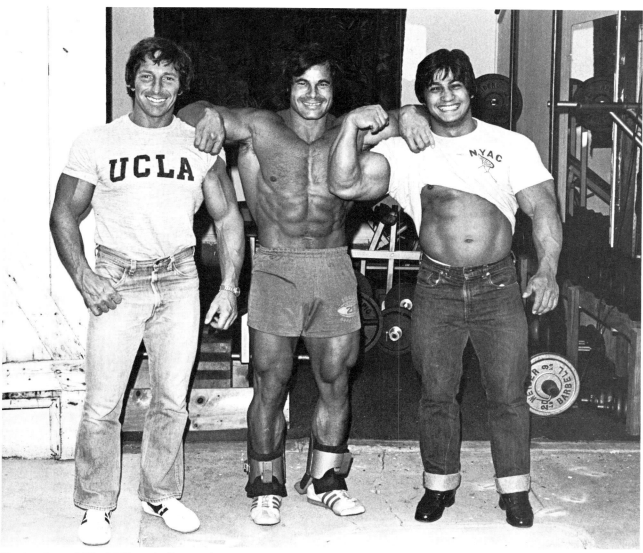

Having fun at World Gym in the early years.

stimulation of exercise will cause an increase in body size. And because the bones are still soft, they can be "stretched" by certain exercises. For example, by doing wide-grip chins or lat-machine pulldowns, your shoulder scapulae are pulled out, making your shoulders wider. And by doing pullovers, you can enlarge your rib-cage, making your chest deeper and bigger. I would recommend a three-day-a-week schedule, training your whole body each session, and doing just one basic exercise per body part, for two or three sets of 10–12 reps. A sample routine might be:

1. Breathing squat, 2 × 15–20 (supersetted) with straight-arm barbell pullovers, 2 × 20
2. Bench press, 3 × 10
3. Wide-grip lat-machine pulldown, 3 × 12
4. Seated wide-grip behind-neck press, 3 × 10
5. Upright row, 2 × 10
6. Deadlift, 2 × 10
7. Barbell Curl, 3 × 10
8. Lying triceps extensions, 3 × 12
9. Wrist curl, 2 × 20
10. Calf raise, 3 × 15
11. Crunch, 3 × 15

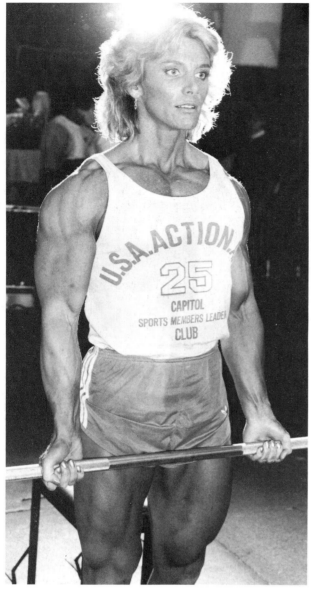

Bev Francis.

CELLULITE

Q I have cellulite on my upper thighs and buttocks. Although my husband does like dimples, he prefers only the ones on my facial cheeks. What do you suggest I do?

A That dimpled, saggy, orange-peel appearance on the hips and upper thighs of many women, usually referred to as cellulite, is actually nothing more, or less than FAT. Double-blind studies of biopsies of cellulite fat and more normal looking fat in the same areas revealed that there is no difference in the chemical makeup of the respective fat cells. The researchers theorized that the difference in appearance of the fat in women with cellulite is likely due to the greater size of the fat cells in these women, which causes local fat stores to bulge and produce the dimpled appearance. A diet to lower your body's overall fat content will be necessary. So reduce your daily calories intake by 500–750 calories. Reducing intake less than 500 calories will not result in any meaningful fat loss, while reducing it more than 750 calories will most assuredly lead to the loss of muscle tissue. Be sure your reduced-calorie diet is well balanced, with portions that include 60 percent carbohydrates, 25 percent protein, and 15 percent fats.

MORE DRUGS!

Q I am a competitive bodybuilder and have won some titles, but only at the state level. To tell you the truth, I am scared that if drug testing comes into force, I will not be able to win. I have heard that HGH (human growth hormone) cannot be detected by any tests. Is this true?

A Human growth hormone is produced naturally by the pituitary gland. When prescribed it is injected, and there is no way at present to detect it. Sometimes L-dopa is taken with HGH to enhance the overall effect. If you want to Frankenstein your looks with acromegaly, to build up your forehead, lengthen your chin, elongate your elbows, and widen your jaw (to the extent that your teeth part in the middle), and increase the likelihood of heart attack and death before the age of 45, then take HGH. A six-week supply will cost only upward of $800. Forget all steroids, my friend. You're just a misguided bodybuilder who wants a short cut to a twenty-dollar trophy and what you perceive as bodybuilding superstar status.

KNEE PROBLEMS

Q I use the Nautilus leg-extension machine and I also perform squats for my legs, but now after several years of training I have very sore knees. Lately I have taken up cross-country running (twice weekly) because I am anxious to keep my legs strong, but my sore knees are making workouts difficult. Any advice is appreciated.

A It seems to me that you have inherited a potential for sore knees. On top of that, you are doing everything possible to make the condition worse. Nautilus leg extensions can prove hard on the knees (especially if there is a tendency to trouble) because the movement starts from an angle at which the feet are well back from the knees. This position can aggravate a weak condition.

Squats, too, may not be for you—especially if you are squatting deep. Certainly your idea of cross-country running is asking for trouble because the rough terrain can aggravate the condition.

I would suggest you take a week or two off from direct leg training. Perform three to four sets of warm-up squats before piling on the weight. Do not squat all the way down; stop just short of going to the parallel position. Keep your feet fairly close together, 12–15 inches, toes slightly pointed outward. After your squats move to either hack lifts or leg presses, but be guided by the comfort of the movement.

If there is any pain or discomfort, you will have to drop these exercises, too. A possible way of getting around sore knees is to perform your leg exercises with much lighter weights, but using many more repetitions. Sets of 40, 50, or even 60 reps can still give great results, while alleviating the knees of excessive strain.

METABOLISM

Q I keep hearing so much about metabolism nowadays. I really don't know what it is or how it works. I am writing to you because I do not want to ask other people for fear of being seen as stupid.

A Metabolism is the rate at which your body burns up energy. It's a burning process similar to that of a lit candle. The

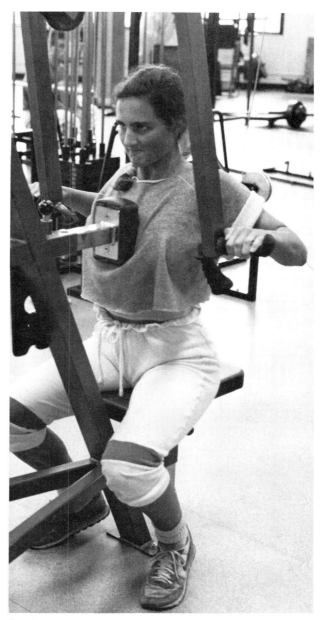

Seated machine rows by Shawn Stouffer.

process consumes oxygen, heat is generated, and carbon dioxide is given off.

Many influences affect the metabolism, stimulating or suppressing it. Thyroid hormones, for example, stimulate the metabolic rate by promoting the production of heat. An episode of vigorous physical activity can increase the metabolic rate. (I have often advocated high-rep squats to speed up the metabolism.) Those who train regularly and vigorously not only tend to increase their metabolic rate during the workout itself, but there is a resid-

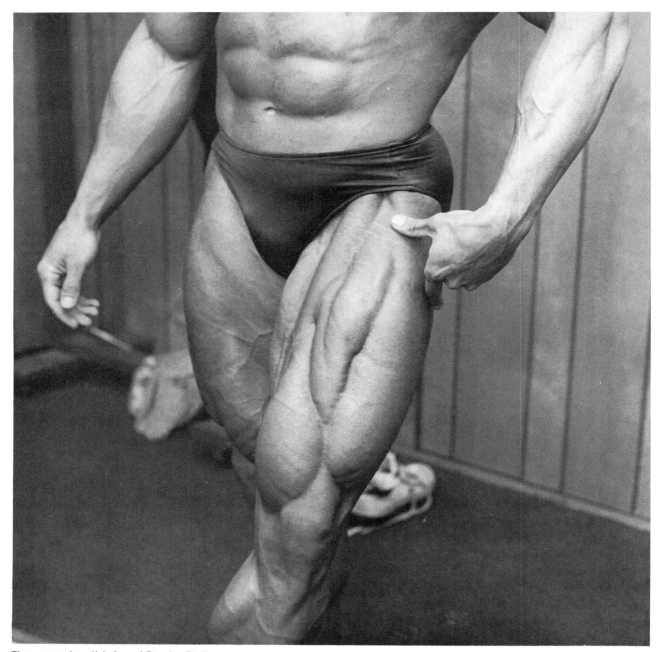

The amazing thighs of Rocky DeFerro.

ual effect for one or two days afterward. You can easily see the benefits of daily training for someone with a sluggish metabolism, especially someone who wishes to lose body fat.

Also the time of day you train is important. Exercising in the morning burns more body fat (up to 70 percent of your calories from stored fat as opposed to 40 percent if you train at night).

PEAK

Q Can you suggest an alternative to one-arm concentration dumbbell curls for developing biceps peak? I have difficulty getting the proper feel with the movement.

A You could try steep-angle (90 degrees) one-arm dumbbell or cable preacher curls. Cable curls, tensing hard at the top, are also excellent, as are bent-over barbell concentration curls (a Robby Robinson favorite). One of the best biceps peakers that is easy to get the proper feel for is lat-machine pulldown curls. Lie on a flat bench placed under a lat-machine bar with your head directly under the bar. Keeping your elbows pointing straight up, grab the bar with a six- to twelve-inch grip and curl it down to your neck in a wide, semicircular arc. Tense your biceps hard for several seconds to get an intense contraction. If you do it properly, you should experience a cramped, knotted feeling. Try three to four sets of 10–15 reps for a better peak. Do not use a lot of weight in this exercise.

NO MORE BI-LATS!

Q I have a problem with my lats. Every time I work them my biceps blow up and hurt. I just can't get my lats to feel *any* exercise. I perform chins, cable rows, pulldowns, rowing, and all I get is a biceps pump and zilch in my lats. I must be doing something wrong, but I don't know what. Are there any pointers or special techniques to solve my problem?

A The lats are difficult to isolate. The only exercise I know that does it is the one Bob Kennedy invented when searching for an ideal combination (isolation and compound) for his preexhaust course. It is the parallel-bar shrug. Adopt a position on the parallel bars with your arms straight and your legs bent under your body or hanging straight down. While maintaining this basic position, bring your shoulders up to your ears (shrug) and then lower them as far as possible (so that the clavicles are as horizontal as they can be). Do 10–15 repetitions. As you get used to this exercise you will have to add resistance in the form of a weight hanging from your hips.

An exercise that almost isolates the lats is the parallel-handle bar pulldowns. Since your biceps are closely involved in most lat exercises, and because they are smaller and weaker than the lats, they can sometimes get in the way. Often they tire

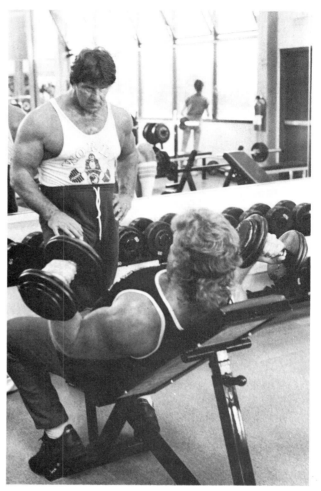

Reg Park provides invaluable advice to those who train at World.

first and prevent you from working the lats hard. To get around the problem, the parallel-handle lat machine's attachment bar (usually only about 22–25 inches long) will help "take out" the biceps and enable you to concentrate on your lat work.

Finally, bear in mind that you can "think" the action into the lats merely by concentrating and conceptualizing the effort into the area.

CUTTING THIGHS

Q I can't cut my legs up, especially near the knee. I train on a three-day-on, one-day-off program (two body parts per workout) and I include squats, lunges, and thigh extensions in my training, but my thighs look blocky, and the skin seems thicker on my thighs than anywhere else. I need your advice.

A Bodybuilders with powerlifter's thighs are not uncommon. Many champion muscle men solved this problem by taking drugs (hormones) and dieting. But I definitely do not recommend this procedure. I'm just relating the facts, that many "thick-skinned" bodybuilders did obtain the cut-up look with drugs.

The natural bodybuilder will find the problem a little tougher to beat. Be strict about your diet. Cut out all whole milk and related products. Cut your foods fat content way down (fat makes you fat). Eat natural, unprocessed foods. No junk. Train your legs with at least one isolation movement each leg workout (thigh extensions, hack machine, sissy squats, Roman chair squats). Pose your thighs every day for five to ten minutes. Learn to control the muscles of each leg in a variety of positions. Make a point of cutting up once a year, whether you are entering a competition or not! Zane does this, and it is important—take a good amino acid supplement.

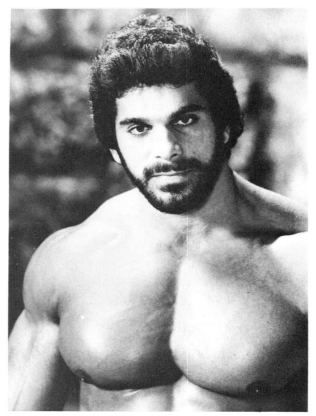

Lou Ferrigno's herculean proportions.

NO TIME TO WASTE

Q I want to know what is the best, truly scientific knowledge in bodybuilding today. I do not want to waste time. Please tell me the best high-tech machinery to use and the best scientific food combinations. I only want to train according to the findings of medical science.

A I'm afraid that science hasn't caught up to the practicing bodybuilder yet. Most champions get to the top by trial and error, not by following scientific findings. Some day science may be able to give us superior machines and nutritional advice, but this is still in the future. Currently science tells us that squats are bad, that nine out of ten medical studies show steroids don't aid muscle growth, that increasing intensity is the only way to larger muscles—but we know differently.

You can put scientific data to use in designing an exercise machine with a cam that exactly corresponds to the strength curve of a particular muscle, but it doesn't amount to a hill of beans to the free-weight bodybuilder who makes better progress using old-fashioned barbells and dumbbells.

Science produced compounds to increase the metabolic rate, but they shut down your thyroid. Science developed advanced steroids, but you end up with internal problems and bitch-tits. Science gave us personalized computer routines that paid out zero dividends. Science gave us hair analysis and body fat tests that vary embarrassingly. As I said, it will come. But don't hold your breath. Science has helped humanity in many ways, but when it comes to bodybuilding it has only served to screw things up.

BIG LOU!

Q I am a fan of the Hulk. And I'm not talking about wrestling's Hulk Hogan. Lou Ferrigno is my man. I want to be just like him. When I saw his body in his Hercules movie I couldn't believe my eyes. I watched him train at World Gym in California, but didn't have the nerve to go up and talk to him. I am particularly interested in his supplemental program. Please let me know what vitamins, etc., Lou takes to keep his body in such great shape.

A At last reckoning Lou took the following supplements daily:

1. One multivitamin pack
2. Mineral tablets
3. Vitamin E (1,000 IU)
4. Bio C
5. Fergon
6. B-complex

FIBER

Q All this talk about fiber in the diet—I just don't know how or where to get the stuff, or even what it is! I train hard four days a week and eat plenty of eggs, but all I read about is fiber. Please put me straight on this matter.

A Fiber is the casing of fruits and vegetables, or the husks of cereals. Fiber has no nutritive value; a deficiency will not cause disease in the sense that too little vitamin C will cause scurvy and even death. During the last century, fiber was systematically removed by the milling process that refined flour, by the canning industry, and by the refinement and overprocessing of most other foods. Fiber is

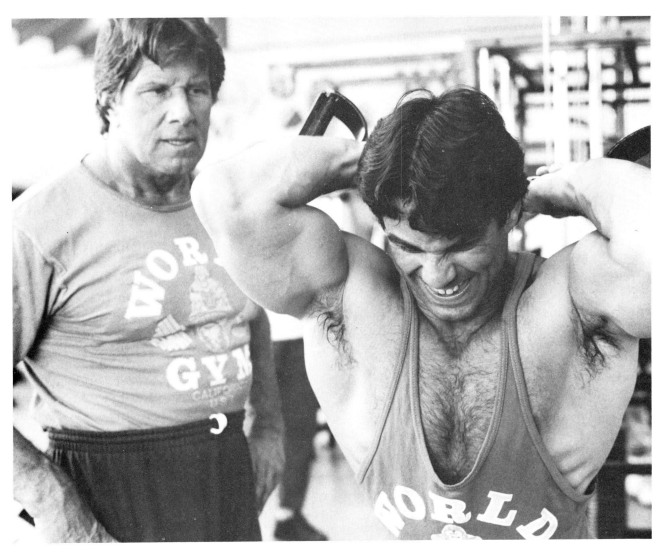

The immortal Reg Park watching his son Jon-Jon perform cable presses.

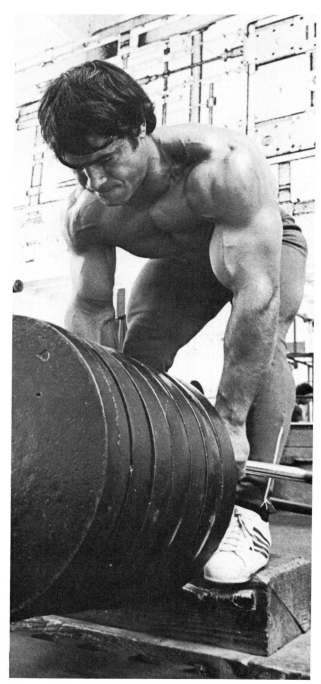

Franco Columbu likes to use extremely heavy weights to build his back.

present in many natural foods, so for the most part try to stay clear of packaged, canned, or processed foods. Eat whole-grain breads, potatoes (not the instant variety), and fresh fruits and vegetables. Bran has the highest fiber content (almost 45 percent), but for optimum health you should get fiber from different sources, including grain, fruits, and vegetables.

Yes, fiber is necessary in the diet. It keeps food passing through the system in a steady, controlled fashion, and helps control blood pressure, diabetes, hemorrhoids, and varicose veins, and it may even help prevent heart problems. All of these benefits help maximize fitness, which in turn will help maximize your bodybuilding progress. Fiber is important.

HEAT BELTS

Q Do heat belts help reduce the stomach?

A Heat belts do not help increase burning of fat to any great extent, but they do help you lose excess water because they greatly increase sweating in the waist area. When combined with exercise and diet, heat belts do create greater losses than diet and exercise alone, but only slightly. One value of heat belts is that they provide support and keep the lower back warm, thus helping to prevent injury, when doing exercises such as squats, overhead presses, deadlifts, and bent rows.

TRAPS

Q I have a long skinny neck and fairly broad shoulders. My big problem is my "traps." I have included heavy deadlifts, cleans, and even upright rowing in my routine, but I just can't fill in my trap area.

A You seem to be neglecting the best direct trapezius exercise of all—shrugs. You can do these with a barbell held in front or behind your hips. Some people prefer dumbbells or even a Universal machine. You could use the standing calf machine. I suggest you start with three sets of 8–10 reps and work up until you are doing six to eight sets of 8–12 reps. Attempt to touch your ears with your shoulders, holding the resistance in the arms-down position. Traps usually grow rapidly once they are subjected to regular progressive-resistance exercise.

REAR HEAD TRICEPS

Q How do you build the part of the triceps right at the back of the arm (I guess it's called the rear head of the triceps)? I just cannot get that area to grow. What should I be doing, and what are the best exercises for that area?

A You may be weak genetically in that area, which could account for the lack of muscle there. By that I mean you may not have a lot of muscle cells to build up in that area, but you should give it a good try anyway. It could be that your lack of growth is due to lack of work. The best exercises for the rear head of the triceps are: kickbacks (raise the dumbbell as high as possible and hold for a count of two, to really give the rear head a good contraction), dips (keep the body upright and lock out hard in the fully contracted position), triceps dips (again, lock out hard and hold at the top in the fully contracted position), and reverse-grip bench presses (best done on a Smith machine because the movement is more concentrated, but it can be done with a barbell, too). On the reverse-grip bench presses, again lock out hard at the top to really put the stress on the rear head. Do one exercise hard for four sets and then superset two of the other suggested exercises. For example, try this routine: weighted dips, 4×8–10; kickbacks, 3×8–10; reverse-grip bench presses, 3–4×6–10; superset triceps dips, 4×12–15. Try putting a plate across your lap to make the triceps dips harder. Concentrate your effort on the rear head, and do the above routine for six weeks. Don't forget to eat well, too, and take your supplements. Diet is the difference between success and failure.

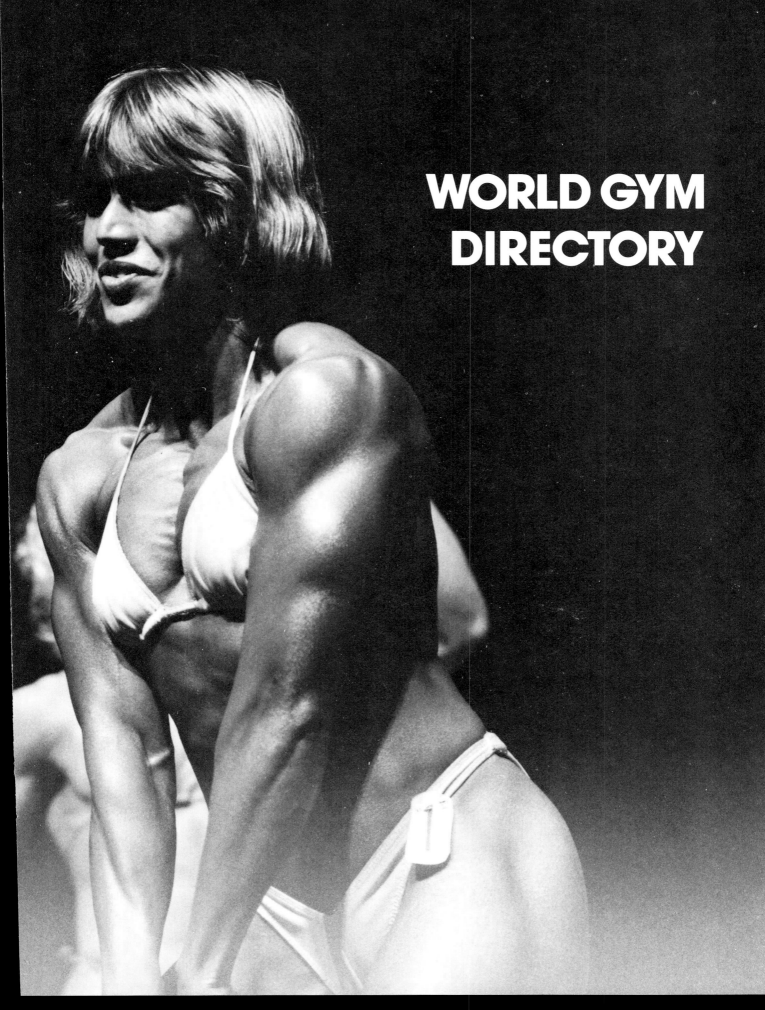

WORLD GYM
DIRECTORY

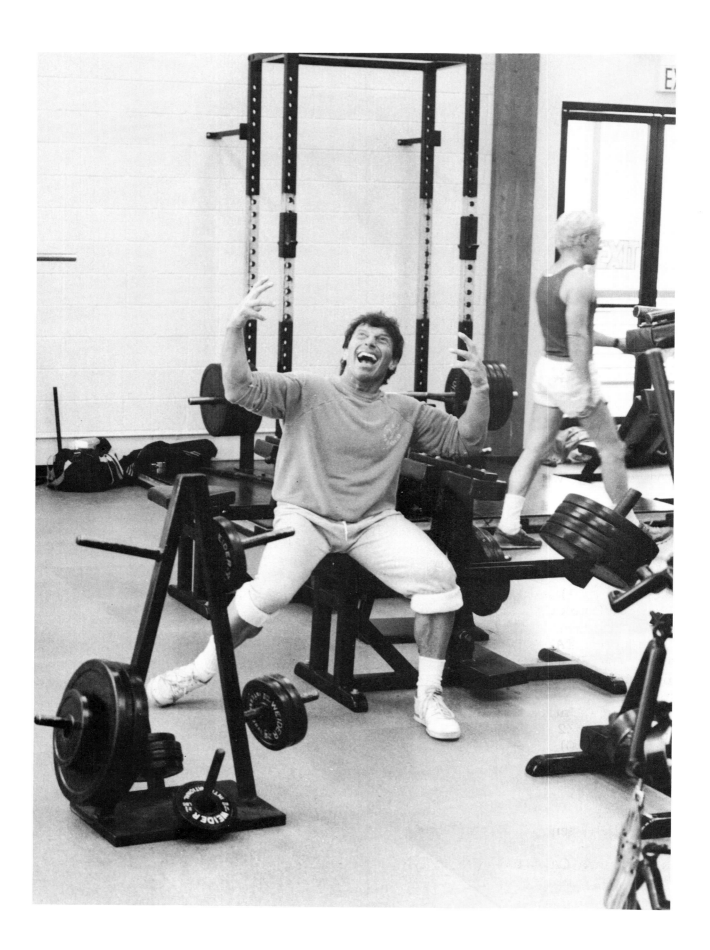

WORLD GYM
DISTRIBUTORS

AUSTRIA: See Germany

AUSTRALIA:
Tropicana
382 Newcastle St.,
Perth, Australia
Attention: Mike Wynn

BELGIUM:
Frank's Health Products P.V.B.A.
De Bosschaertstraat 142
2020 Antwerpen - Keil
Belgium
Telephone: (301) 16.21.81
Attention: Frank Gall

CANADA and EASTERN U.S.:
Body Sports Promotions
3663 Mavis Road
Unit #15
Mississauga, Ontario
Canada L5C 2Z2
Telephone: (800) 387-9497 or
(416) 273-3906
Attention: Robert Gallop

DENMARK:
Sven-Ole Thorsen
P.O. Box 1688
Santa Monica, CA 90406

ENGLAND/U.K.:
Tropicana
Unit 4, Aston Cross Estate,
53 Litchfield Road
Birmingham B6
England
Attention: D.E. McInerney
Telephone: (021) 326-8311

FRANCE and ITALY:
Franco Fassi
Fassi Sport Spa,
Strada Francesca N.42
24040 Zingiona (Bergamo)
Italia
Telephone: 035/885034

GERMANY:
Ludwig Brummer Import GMBH
Lindwurmstrasse 125-127
8000 München 2
Postfach 15 03 40
West Germany

HAWAII:
World Gym Maui
1325 So. Kihei Road
Kihei, Maui,
HI 96753
Telephone: (808) 874-0101
Attention: Elliott Cuvin

SOUTH AFRICA:
World Gym South Africa
Reg Park and Jon-Jon Park
P.O. Box 32370
Braaamfontein 2017
Transvaal, South Africa

UNITED STATES:
World Gym Venice
c/o Ace Trophy
609 Rose Ave.
Venice, CA 90291
Telephone: (213) 399-6290
Attention: Steve Tanchuck

WORLD GYM LOCATIONS

Canadian Affiliates
ALBERTA:
World Gym Calgary
105 58th Avenue S.E.
Calgary, Alberta
Canada T2H ON8
Telephone: (403) 258-0820
Attention: Rob Leach

World Gym
771 Northmount Drive
Northwest Calgary, Alberta
Canada T2L 0A1
Telephone: (403) 284-4597
Attention: Rob Leach

WINNIPEG:
World Gym
413 McPhillips Street
Winnipeg, Manitoba
Canada R2X 2Z8
(204) 586-8005
Attention: David Glass

ONTARIO:
World Gym
909 Pape Avenue
Toronto, Ontario
Canada M4K 3V1
(416) 469-4184

QUEBEC:
World Gym Laval
Serge Fournier
2514 Boul. Le Corbusier
Laval, Quebec
Canada H7S 2H2
Attention: Andre Elie

World Gym Longueuil
15 Prevost
Longueuil, Quebec
Canada
(514) 679-2508
Attention: Tony Fragiskos

World Gym Montreal
800 Boul. de Maisonneuve E.,
Suite 201
Place Dupuis,
Montreal, Quebec
Canada H2L 4L8
(514) 729-6704
Attention: Andre Elie

World Gym Quebec City
Messrs. Cashman, Kadri & Sonsouy
c/o Bruce Cashman
117 de la Rivière
St. Nicholas
P.Q., Canada G0S 2Z0
(418) 659-3463

SASKATCHEWAN:
World Gym Regina - 2 Locations
4025 Albert Street
Regina, Saskatchewan
Canada S4S 3R6

10 - Hesse Bay
Regina, Saskatchewan
Canada S4R 7Z9
(306) 545-5944
Attention: Rose Turner

United States Affiliates:
ARIZONA:
World Fitness Center
2713 W. Northern Avenue
Phoenix, AZ 85051
(602) 864-1604
Attention: Steven & David Reiter

World Gym Scotsdale
1465 N. Hayden Road
Scotsdale, AZ 85257
(602) 252-0366
Attention: Cindy & Dennis Goldberg

CALIFORNIA:
World Gym Bakersfield
4101 Easton Drive
Bakersfield, CA 93309
Attention: Phil Robb

World Gym Ontario
2242 Euclid, Suites A-J
Ontario, CA 91761
(714) 861-2226 - GYM
Attention: David Dexheimer/
    Kimberly Clark

World Gym Escondido
1872 E. Valley Parkway
Escondido, CA 92027
(619) 489-8267
Attention: Jonathan and C.J.

World Gym Lodi
1030 S. Hutchings
Lodi, CA 95240
(209) 333-7447
Attention: Kevin Kendrick

World Gym Manteca
965 E. Yosemite
Manteca, CA 95336
(209) 823-8285
Attention: Mike Stevens & Russ Kuhn

World Gym Marin County
941 Sir Francis Drake Blvd.
Kentfield, CA 94904
(415) 453-2300
Attention: John Gorgot

World Gym Modesto
3500 Coffee Road
Modesto, CA 95353
(209) 529-BODY
Attention: Mike Stevens & Russ Kuhn

World Gym - San Diego/Clairemont Mesa
3968 Clairemont Mesa Blvd.
San Diego, CA 92117
(619) 483-9100
Attention: Jim, Mara & Mae Della Valle

World Gym North Stockton
2233 Grand Canal Blvd., #214
Stockton, CA 95207
(209) 474-8822
Attention: Kevin Kendrick

World Gym Roseville
212 F. Harding Plaza
Roseville, CA 95678
(916) 781-2990 gym
Attention: George F. Hillenbrand

World Gym San Jose
Martin Lingle
Gordon Balena
P.O. Box 10323
San Jose, CA 95157
(408) 238-4333

World Gym Woodland Hills
23210 Ventura Blvd.
Woodland Hills, CA 91364
(818) 99-WORLD
Attention: Kyle Betton, Wendy Betton,
    and Steven L. Buckingham (Buck)

COLORADO:
World Gym Aurora
14080 E. Alameda
Aurora, CO 80012
(303) 773-1121
Attention: Jay Kee Jacobson

World Gym Denver
3124 W. 34th Avenue
Denver, CO 80211
(303) 455-9106
Attention: Craig Elliott

World Gym Littleton
7562 S. University Blvd.
Littleton, CO 80122
(303) 796-9231
Attention: Brian Greenhouse

FLORIDA:
World Gym Ft. Lauderdale
1119 North Federal Highway
Fort Lauderdale, FL
(718) 639-0340
Attention: Joseph Robson

HAWAII:
World Gym Maui
1325 So. Kihei Road
Kihei, Maui,
HI 96753
(808) 874-0101
Attention: Elliott Cuvin

World Gym
1701 Ala Wai Blvd.
Honolulu, HI 92815
(808) 942-8171
Attention: Mr. Harold Mathews

KENTUCKY:
World Gym Louisville
4160 Bardstown Road
Louisville, KY 40218
(502) 499-7476 or 499-7474
Attention: Danny Corrigan

MARYLAND:
World Gym Baltimore
World Gym & Fitness Center Inc.
7739 Eastpoint Mall
Baltimore, MD 21224
(301) 288-2639
Attention: Keith Vasquez

World Gym Wheaton Plaza
11160 Veirs Mill Road
Wheaton, MD 20902
(301) 949-8000/G
Attention: Pete Heon

MASSACHUSETTS:
World Gym Newton/Waltham
385 California Street
Newton, MA 02158
(617) 965-3561
Attention: Joseph M. Rizzo

World Gym Somerville
c/o Kevin Lavelle
25 Grant Street
Waltham, MA 02154
Kevin at work:
(617) 633-3707 or (617) 923-5131
Attention: Leonard P. Cuzzupe,
   Vice President
(Cuzzupe, Lima, Correia & Litman)

NEW JERSEY:
World Gym
1214 North Black Horse Pike
Glendora, NJ 08029
(609) 939-9846
Attention: Ralph Pepino

World Gym - Middlesex
472 Lincoln Blvd.
Middlesex, NJ 08901
(201) 356-9836 or (201) 752-5509 HM
Attention: Adam Salamon

World Gym Red Bank
129 Monmouth Street
Red Bank, NJ 07701
(201) 530-3666
Attention: John Braycewski

NEW YORK:
World Gym Buffalo
2525 Walden Avenue
Cheektowaga, NY 14225
(716) 683-9852
Attention: Chris Reichart

World Gym Queens
7402 Eliot
Middlevillage, NY 11379
(718) 426-9869
Attention: Tony Schetinno

World Gym of Medford
2609C Route 112
Medford, NY 11763
(516) 361-9437
Attention: Steve Weiner

NORTH CAROLINA:
World Gym Raleigh
David Gillespie
6704 Old Wake Forrest Road
Raleigh, NC 27604

OHIO:
World Gym Cincinnati
4766 Dues Drive
Cincinnati, OH 45246
(513) 874-8384

World Gym Columbus
James Lorimer
Robert C. Lorimer
Mitchell Adams
7535 Pingue Drive
Columbus, OH
(614) 431-9999

World Gym Macedonia
7792 Capital Blvd.
Macedonia, OH 44056
(216) 467-4469
Attention: John Kleban & John Palsa

World Gym Lake County
P.O. Box 1073
Mentor, OH 44060
(216) 953-9753
Attention: Kaminski & Bouffard

TEXAS:
World Gym Abilene
3202D N. 1st
Abilene, TX 79603
(915) 672-7997
Attention: Kenneth G. Lain

WASHINGTON:
World Gym Lynnwood
Josh Fallis
18905-33rd Avenue W.
Lynnwood, WA 98036
(206) 775-8442

WEST VIRGINIA:
World Gym Charleston
3200 Chesterfield Avenue
Charleston, WV 25344
(304) 346-2801
Attention: Ray Wiley

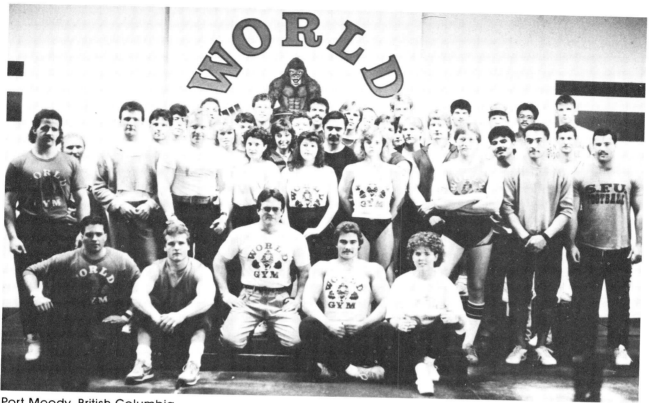

Port Moody, British Columbia.

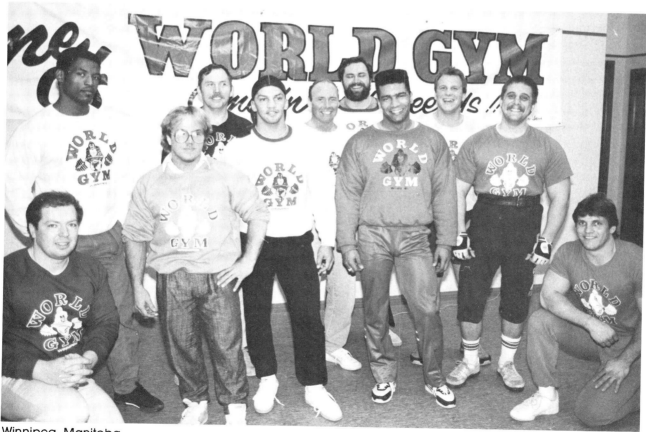

Winnipeg, Manitoba.

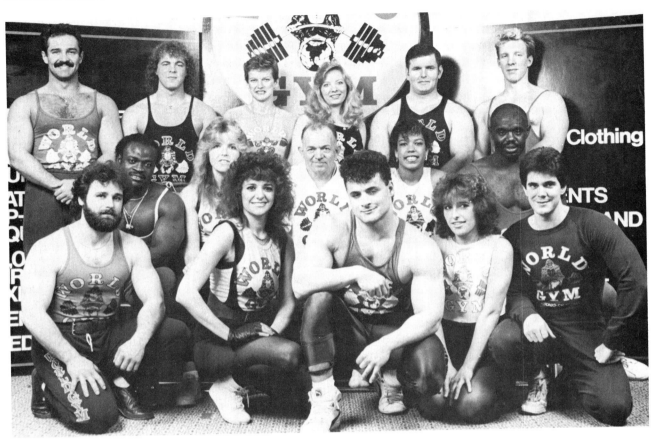

Toronto, Canada.

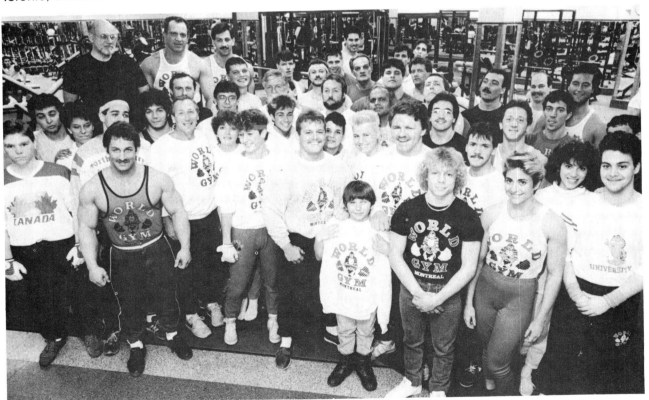

Montreal, Quebec.

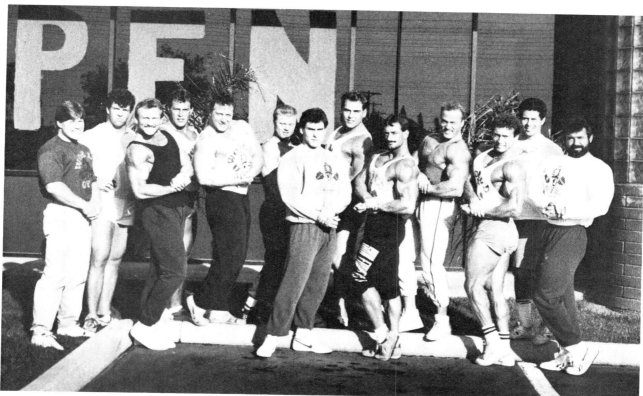

Scotsdale, Arizona.

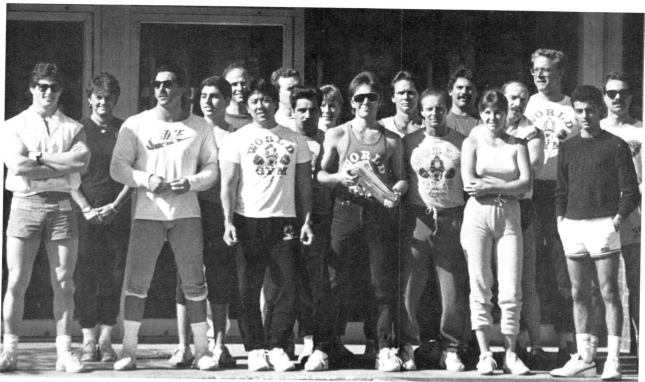

Kentfield, California.

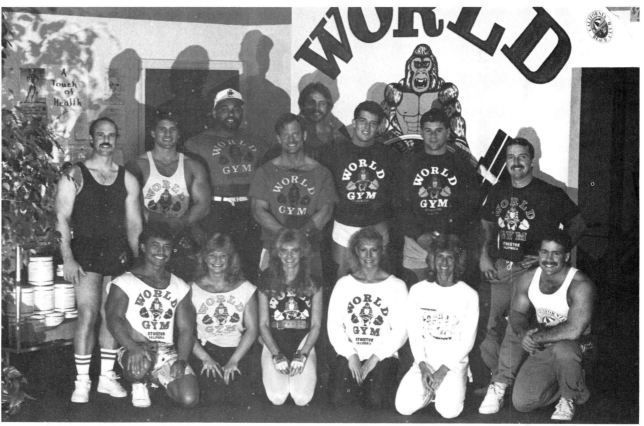

Stockton, California.

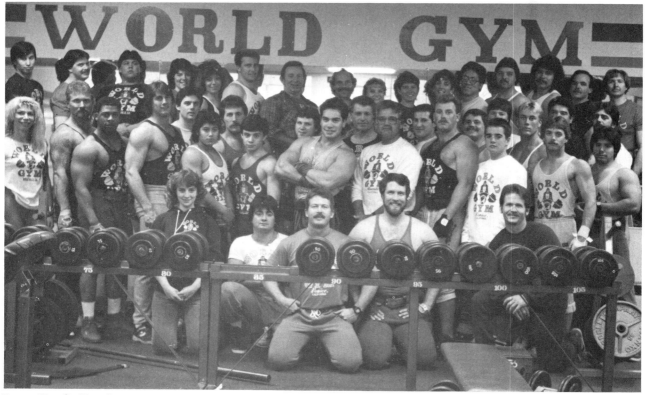

Roseville, California.

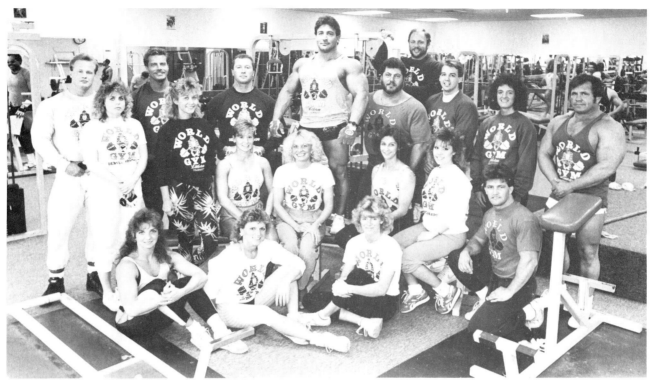

Littleton, Colorado.

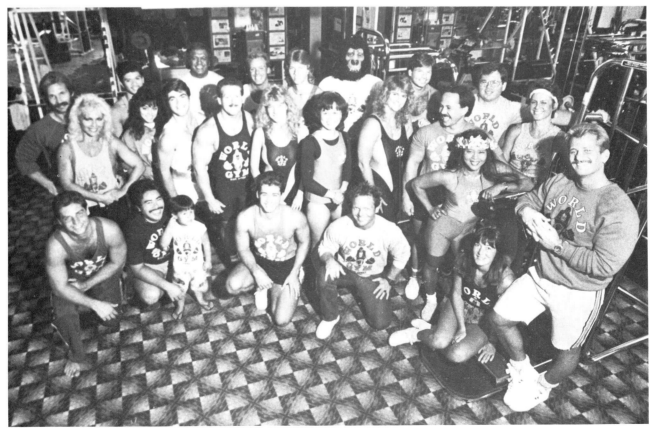

Kihie, Hawaii.

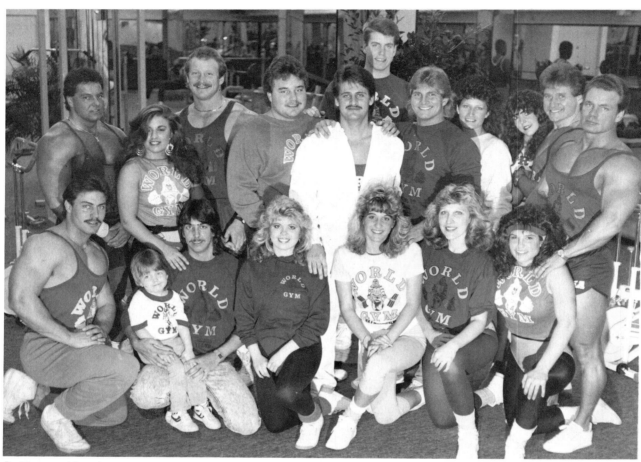

Baltimore, Maryland.

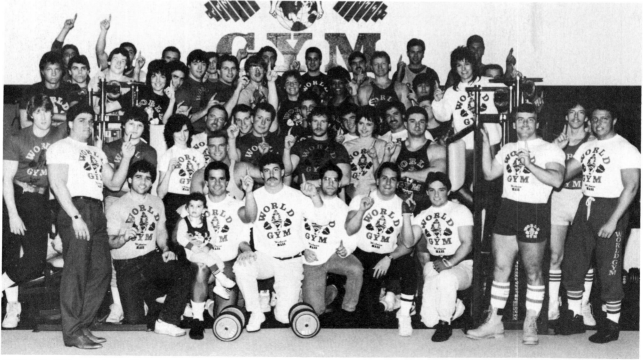

Wobrun, Massachusetts.

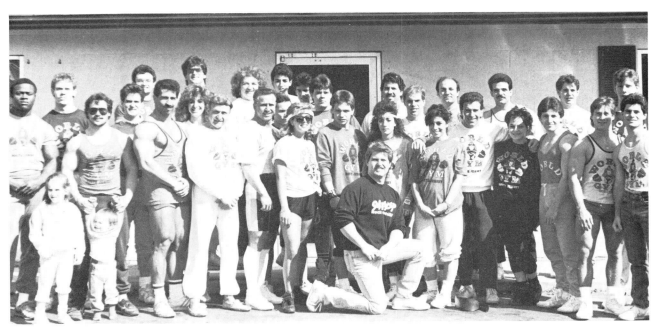

Glendora, New Jersey.

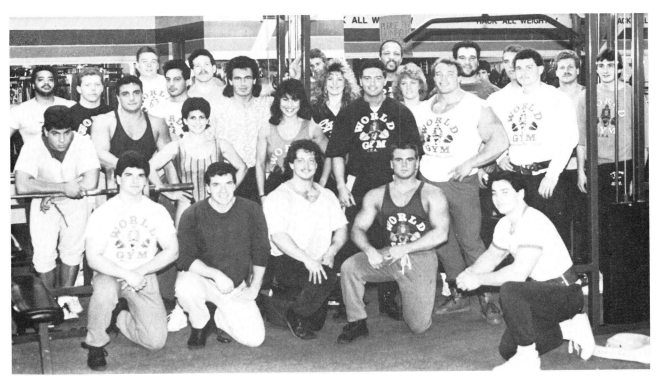

Middlesex, New Jersey.

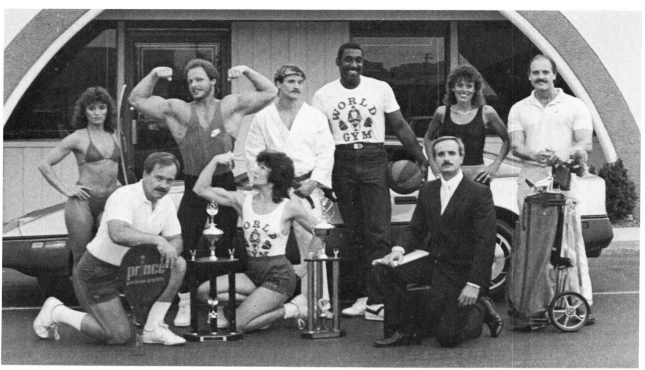

Cincinnati, Ohio.

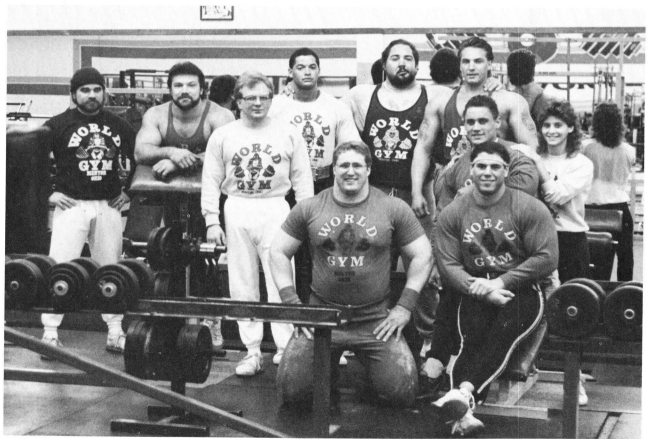

Mentor, Ohio.

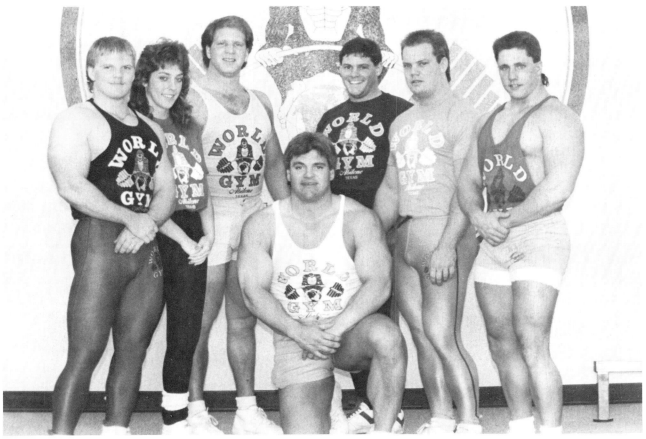

Abilene, Texas.

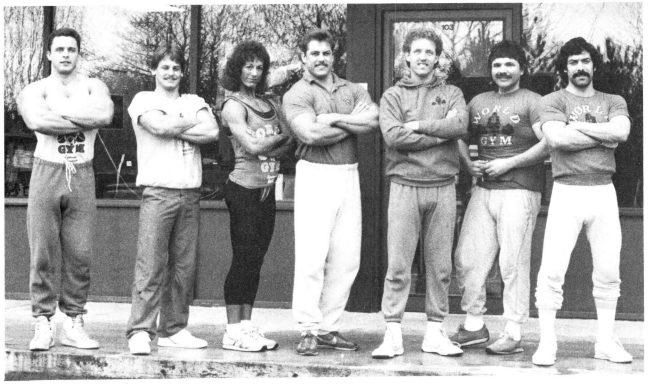

Lynnwood, Washington.

INDEX